Hysterectomy

CURRENT TOPICS IN OBSTETRICS AND GYNECOLOGY

Series Editor
Morton A. Stenchever, MD
Professor and Chairman
Department of Obstetrics and Gynecology
University of Washington
School of Medicine
Seattle, Washington

Controversies in Reproductive Endocrinology and Infertility
Michael R. Soules, MD

Caring for the Older Woman
Morton A. Stenchever, MD, and George A. Aagaard, MD

Caring for the Exercising Woman
Ralph W. Hale, MD

Gynecologic Oncology: Treatment Rationale and Techniques
Benjamin E. Greer, MD, and Jonathan S. Berek, MD

Obstetrics: Psychological and Psychiatric Syndromes
John Patrick O'Grady, MD

Infections and Abortion
Sebastian Faro, MD, and Mark Pearlman, MD

Hysterectomy
Thomas G. Stovall, MD

Hysterectomy

Edited by

Thomas G. Stovall, MD
Associate Professor
Head, Section of Gynecology
Department of Obstetrics and Gynecology
Wake Forest University/
The Bowman Gray School of Medicine
Winston-Salem, North Carolina

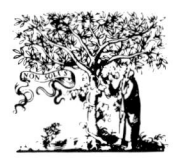

Elsevier
New York • Amsterdam • London • Tokyo

No responsibility is assumed by the Publisher for any injury and/or damage to persons or property as a matter of products liability, negligence, or otherwise, or from any use or operation of any methods, products, instructions, or ideas contained in the material herein. No suggested test or procedure should be carried out unless, in the reader's judgment, its risk is justified. Because of rapid advances in the medical science, we recommend that the independent verification of diagnoses and drug dosages should be made. Discussion, views, and recommendations as to medical procedures, choice of drugs, and drug dosages are the the responsibility of the authors.

Elsevier Science Publishing Co., Inc.
655 Avenue of the Americas, New York, New York 10010

Sole distributors outside the United States and Canada:
Elsevier Science Publishers B.V.
P.O. Box 211, 1000 AE Amsterdam, The Netherlands

© 1993 by Elsevier Science Publishing Co., Inc.

This book has been registered with the Copyright Clearance Center, Inc. For further information, please contact the Copyright Clearance Center, Inc., Salem, Massachusetts.

All inquiries regarding copyrighted material from this publication, other than reproduction through the Copyright Clearance Center, Inc., should be directed to: Rights and Permissions Department, Elsevier Science Publishing Co., 655 Avenue of the Americas, New York, New York 10010. FAX 212-633-3977.

This book is printed on acid-free paper.

Library of Congress Cataloging-in-Publication Data

Hysterectomy / edited by Thomas G. Stovall.
    p.   cm.—(Current topics in obstetrics and gynecology)
  Includes index.
  ISBN 0-444-01664-3 (hardcover : alk. paper)
  1. Hysterectomy. I. Stovall, Thomas G. II. Series.
  [DNLM: 1. Hysterectomy. WP 660 H999]
RG391.H98 1993
618.1′453—dc20
DNLM/DLC
for Library of Congress   92-49172
                                              CIP

Current Printing (last digit):
10 9 8 7 6 5 4 3 2 1

Manufactured in the United States of America

Contents

Foreword / vii

Preface / ix

Contributors / xi

Chapter **1**
Preoperative Considerations for Hysterectomy / 1
Elisabeth H. Quint, MD, and Thomas E. Elkins, MD

Chapter **2**
Current Indications for Hysterectomy / 17
M. Chrystie Timmons, MD, and W. Allen Addison, MD

Chapter **3**
Vaginal Versus Abdominal Hysterectomy / 27
David H. Nichols, MD

Chapter **4**
Prophylactic Antibiotic Use with Elective Hysterectomy / 35
David L. Hemsell, MD

Chapter **5**
Urinary and Intestinal Tract Injuries / 51
Donald G. Gallup, MD

Chapter **6**
Management of Intraoperative and Postoperative Hemorrhage at the Time of Hysterectomy / 79
James L. Breen, MD, and John T. Comerci, MD

Chapter 7
Controversial Techniques During Hysterectomy / 103
Thomas G. Stovall, MD

Chapter 8
Additional Surgical Procedures at the Time of Hysterectomy / 115
Robert L. Summit, Jr, MD

Chapter 9
Hysterectomy in the Face of Pelvic Inflammatory Disease / 133
David E. Soper, MD

Chapter 10
Postoperative Care / 147
W. Glenn Hurt, MD

Chapter 11
Psychosocial Aspects of Hysterectomy / 163
Renate H. Rosenthal, PhD, and Frank W. Ling, MD

Chapter 12
Residual Ovarian Disease After Hysterectomy / 183
Raymond A. Lee, MD

Chapter 13
Laparoscopic-Assisted Vaginal Hysterectomy / 191
Thomas G. Stovall, MD, and Robert L. Summitt, Jr, MD

Index / 201

Foreword

During the past century, hysterectomy has become the major surgical procedure performed by gynecologists. Over time, indications for this operation have changed as the pathophysiology of uterine diseases has been better defined and as alternative therapies for many disorders have been developed. In addition, social changes in each decade have affected perceived indications for hysterectomy. Multiple factors are likely to continue to influence the frequency of hysterectomy well into the future.

Dr. Thomas G. Stovall has assembled an outstanding group of pelvic surgeons to address the various aspects of hysterectomy in the 1990s. Within this volume, consideration is given to: current indications; preoperative preparation of the patient; decisions regarding the route of surgery, including new concepts of laparoscopic-assisted hysterectomy; the use of prophylactic antibiotics; and the management of minor, as well as severe, surgical and medical complications. Psychosocial aspects are carefully covered and the significance of residual ovarian disease post-hysterectomy is discussed.

Our series, **Current Topics in Obstetrics and Gynecology**, has attempted to present important new or changing and/or controversial areas of the specialty of Obstetrics and Gynecology. *Hysterectomy* is a worthwhile addition to our list; it is consistent with our goals for the series. Indeed, this book should be required reading for all gynecologists, whether they are newly entering the field or have been practicing for several years, since it offers an up-to-date, timely discussion of a major topic within our specialty.

Morton A. Stenchever, MD

Preface

Over 400 years have passed since the first successful hysterectomy was recorded. During the last 100 years, volumes of literature have accumulated on specific technical aspects of vaginal and abdominal hysterectomy, operative indications have been proposed, and intraoperative and postoperative complications discussed. The morbidity associated with hysterectomy has been greatly reduced with refinement of gynecologic surgical techniques, effective antibiotic prophylaxis, improved surgical training, and the development of improved suture materials.

The purpose of this volume is to review some of the controversial aspects or issues not frequently discussed regarding hysterectomy. When compiling this book, I asked experts in the field of gynecologic surgery to lend their knowledge to the discussion. Every attempt has been made to provide the most up-to-date and timely information possible, including the potential role of the laparoscopic-assisted vaginal hysterectomy.

Not only do I wish to thank each contributor to this book, but I also wish to say a special word of thanks to my secretary, Hope H. Pittman, for her countless hours in manuscript preparation. It is with a sense of satisfaction that I offer this volume on hysterectomy, and it is my hope that it will be of use to clinicians and teachers as we pursue quality care for our patients.

Thomas G. Stovall, MD

Contributors

W. Allen Addison, MD
Professor and Director, Division of Gynecology, Department of Obstetrics and Gynecology, Duke University Medical Center, Durham, North Carolina

James L. Breen, MD
Professor and Chairman, Department of Obstetrics and Gynecology, Jefferson Medical College, St. Barnabus Medical Center, Livingston, New Jersey

John T. Comerci, MD
Chief Resident, Department of Obstetrics and Gynecology, St. Barnabus Medical Center, Livingston, New Jersey

Thomas E. Elkins, MD
Professor and Chairman, Department of Obstetrics and Gynecology, School of Medicine in New Orleans, Louisiana State University Medical Center, New Orleans, Louisiana

Donald G. Gallup, MD
Professor and Director, Division of Gynecologic Oncology, Department of Obstetrics and Gynecology, Medical College of Georgia, Augusta, Georgia

David L. Hemsell, MD
Professor and Director, Division of Gynecology, Department of Obstetrics and Gynecology, University of Texas, SW Medical Center at Dallas, Dallas, Texas

W. Glenn Hurt, MD
Professor, Department of Obstetrics and Gynecology, Medical College of Virginia, Virginia Commonwealth University, Richmond, Virginia

Raymond A. Lee, MD
Chair, Division of Gynecologic Surgery, and Consultant, Department of Obstetrics and Gynecology and Surgery, Mayo Clinic and Mayo Foundation, Professor of Obstetrics and Gynecology, Mayo Medical School, Rochester, Minnesota

Frank W. Ling, MD
Associate Professor and Director, Division of Gynecology, Department of Obstetrics and Gynecology, University of Tennessee, Memphis, Memphis, Tennessee

David H. Nichols, MD
Professor and Chairman, Department of Obstetrics and Gynecology, Women and Infant's Hospital of Rhode Island, Brown University, Providence, Rhode Island

Elisabeth H. Quint, MD
Lecturer, Department of Obstetrics and Gynecology, University of Michigan Medical School, Ann Arbor, Michigan

Renate Rosenthal, PhD
Associate Professor, Department of Psychiatry, University of Tennessee, Memphis, Memphis, Tennessee

David E. Soper, MD
Associate Professor, Department of Obstetrics and Gynecology, Medical College of Virginia, Virginia Commonwealth University, Richmond, Virginia

Thomas G. Stovall, MD
Associate Professor and Head, Section of Gynecology, Department of Obstetrics and Gynecology, Wake Forest University/The Bowman Gray School of Medicine, Winston-Salem, North Carolina

Robert L. Summitt, Jr, MD
Assistant Professor, Division of Gynecology, Department of Obstetrics and Gynecology, University of Tennessee, Memphis, Memphis, Tennessee

M. Chrystie Timmons, MD
Assistant Professor, Division of Gynecology, Department of Obstetrics and Gynecology, Duke University Medical Center, Durham, North Carolina

Chapter 1

Preoperative Considerations for Hysterectomy

Elisabeth H. Quint, MD, and Thomas E. Elkins, MD

The totality of concerns facing the gynecologic surgeon considering a hysterectomy as a procedure to recommend to a patient, or to undertake as an emergency, go far beyond the limits of this chapter. Although hysterectomy is performed often in the United States, no such procedure should ever be considered "routine" because of the wide variation in patients' medical, psychological, and social situations, which all may impact on the decision to perform a hysterectomy. This chapter seeks only to review selected aspects of preoperative concerns, recognizing that many others may be important in certain instances.

Informed Consent

In 1914, Justice Cardozo pronounced these oft-quoted phrases in a case cited as the "root-premise" of consent law:

Every human being of adult years and sound mind has a right to determine what shall be done with his own body, and a surgeon who performs an operation without his patient's consent commits an assault for which he is liable in damages.[1,2]

Through the 1960s, the benefit of the patient remained the governing principle of health care, despite Justice Cardozo's comments. However, since the 1970s, this concern has been modified to underscore the patient's autonomy in medical decisions. The concept of informed consent clearly defines this change in emphasis.

Informed consent is best understood as a process, or as a conversation, rather than a signed (often preprinted) form. Material elements of informed consent include a description of the procedure and why it is recommended, injuries associated with the procedure, alternatives to the procedure, the projected outcome and relative chances of success for the procedure, and information about the costs for the procedure and aftercare. However, the ethical concepts of informed consent go far beyond these basic elements.

The American College of Obstetricians and Gynecologists Committee on Ethics produced an updated statement on this topic in May 1992, entitled "Ethical Dimensions of Informed Consent."[3] The nine ethical components of informed consent are summarized at the beginning of the document:

1. Informed consent for medical treatment and for participation in medical research is an ethical requirement (which legal doctrines and requirements can in part reflect).
2. Informed consent is an expression of respect for the patient as a person; it particularly respects a patient's moral right to bodily integrity, to reproductive capacities, and to the support of the patient's freedom within caring relationships.
3. Informed consent not only ensures the protection of the patient against unwanted medical treatment, but it also makes possible the active involvement of the patient in her or his medical planning and care.
4. Freedom is maximized in relationships marked by mutuality and equality; this offers both an ethical ideal and an ethical guideline for the physician–patient relationship.
5. Communication is necessary if informed consent is to be realized, and physicians can help to find ways to facilitate communication not only in individual relations with patients but also in the structured context of medical care institutions.
6. Informed consent should be looked on as a process, a process that includes ongoing shared information and developing choices as long as one is seeking medical assistance.
7. The ethical requirement of informed consent need not conflict with physician's overall ethical obligation to a principle of beneficence; that is, every effort should be made to incorporate a commitment to informed consent within a commitment to provide medical benefit to patients and thus to respect them as whole and embodied persons.
8. There are limits to the ethical obligation of informed consent, but a clear justification should be given for any abridgement or suspension of the general obligation.
9. Because ethical requirements and legal requirements cannot be equated, physicians should also acquaint themselves with the legal requirements of informed consent.

The lengthy discussion that follows these nine statements goes beyond this chapter in detail. However, the emphasis on informed consent for the gynecologic surgeon is clear. It is a concept based on thorough patient education, honest communication, and caring trust. The document recognized limitations to complete informed consent in any setting, and the need to allow a broad enough statement of intentions to manage unforeseen findings or complications in surgery. However, this in no way weakens the ethical requirement of informed consent before surgery.

Psychological Aspects of Hysterectomy

Part of the preoperative discussion with patients about hysterectomy should include concerns for the possible psychological effect of hysterectomy. As Freeman noted, all surgeons have seen the emotional cripple after hysterectomy (especially if bilateral salpingo-oophorectomy is included) who (1) feels de-sexed and damaged, (2) complains of continuing pelvic pain without structural cause, (3) no longer has sexual desire, (4) has a dry vagina and whose sexual excitement has vanished, (5) has lost her ability to trust and lives in rage and bitterness, (6) feels old before her time, (7) is abandoned by her lover or drives her lover away, and (8) terminates her sexual identity and begins to draw in the edges of her life.[4] It is important to address a woman's fear of these issues and to be supportive even before surgery occurs.

Roeske has identified 13 factors related to poor prognosis for mental health following hysterectomy: (1) gender identity issues—the hyperfeminine woman copes less well, (2) previous adverse reactions to stress, (3) previous depressive episodes, (4) depression or other mental illness in her family of origin, (5) a history of multiple physical complaints (especially low back pain), (6) numerous hospitalizations and surgeries, (7) age less than 35 at time of hysterectomy, (8) a wish for a child or for more children, (9) anticipations that surgery will produce a loss of interest in and satisfaction from coitus, (10) husband's or significant other's negative attitude toward hysterectomy, (11) marital dissatisfaction and instability, (12) disapproving cultural and religious attitudes, and (13) lack of avocational involvement.[5] Preoperative assessment of these risks should lead physicians to anticipate those patients who may need psychosocial or psychosexual counseling help after surgery.

Often, simply addressing the patient's fears about the psychological effects of surgery serves as the best way of avoiding later psychological damage. This may be as important, in some instances, as the objective, preoperative discussions about the surgical risks of damage to adjacent pelvic and abdominal structures, risks of hemorrhage or infection, and even death rates from surgery or anesthesia, which are all considered routine parts of the informed consent process. The gynecologic surgeon should show special concern for the multiple effects that hysterectomy may have on reproduction, sexuality, self-image, and psychological functioning.

History and Physical Examination

One obvious part of the preoperative assessment of any patient being scheduled for major surgery is the history and physical examination. The scope of this effort goes far beyond the limits of this chapter, so any full discussion is impossible. However, the importance of this part of the preoperative assessment can perhaps best be emphasized by recalling some of the situations in which a careful history and physical examination is a key factor in directing patient care. The person who takes even one or two aspirin tablets daily, or any number of medications that contain aspirin, may not be recognized until the time of postoperative hemorrhage. Prior episodes of postpartum hemorrhage may indicate a need for clotting mechanism assessment as well. Failure to discover familial hyperthermia or food or drug allergies may be lethal. Likewise, overlooking chronic reflux in a patient with hiatal hernia may put the patient at increased risk for aspiration with general anesthesia. Performing a hysterectomy on the anniversary of the death of a spouse may lead to intense posthysterectomy depression.

A careful history and physical examination should make it possible to order preoperative laboratory studies selectively, but with completeness. Intraoperative and postoperative complications may be anticipated much more accurately, thus facilitating more thorough and reasonable informed consent. The history and physical examination is truly an essential part of gynecologic surgery.

Diagnostic Procedures

In general, every effort should be made, within reason, to determine the extent of pelvic pathology prior to hysterectomy with outpatient studies. Pelvic ultrasonography, computerized tomographic scans, and even magnetic resonance imaging studies may be helpful adjuncts to the pelvic examination (but should never be considered total replacements for speculum visualization and bimanual palpation). Cervical cytology should have been noted as negative within 1 year of surgery.

Some still consider an endometrial biopsy to be mandatory before any hysterectomy. In the era of preoperative radiation for endometrial carcinoma, this seemed reasonable. However, now that radiation therapy for endometrial cancer is planned only after evaluation of the entire hysterectomy specimen, endometrial biopsy seems rarely indicated for the sole purpose of preoperative screening. Rather, biopsy (and dilation and curettage) should be done preoperatively in those patients thought to be at significant risk for endometrial carcinoma. These risk factors have been well established, and include unopposed estrogen, menopause after 52 years, obesity, nulliparity, diabetes, feminizing ovarian tumors, polycystic ovarian syndrome, and perhaps radiation therapy. Endometrial sampling just as a preoperative routine is no longer mandatory.

Preoperative testing is used to identify problems or disease processes that may change the surgical procedure, the anesthesia, or the postoperative management of the patient. The determination of which laboratory tests and radiologic studies are necessary prior to hysterectomy depends largely on history, physical examination, and age of the patient, as well as the indication for the procedure. Several tests should be routinely performed in the office prior to hysterectomy. A Papanicolaou smear should be done on every woman and mammography should be performed as indicated by age. A stool guaiac test is performed in all women over the age of 40. All other testing must be evaluated on an individual basis.

Routine screening procedures have been shown to be expensive and not very useful. Kaplan et al stated that, in a review of 2,000 patients undergoing elective surgery, 60% of preoperative testing could have been eliminated.[6] A recent review from the Mayo Clinic found 160 abnormal tests in 3,782 asymptomatic healthy patients.[7] Thirty of these were predictable on the basis of history or physical examination. Only 47 prompted further investigation, and no delay in surgery was necessitated. Their conclusion is that, in healthy patients, no routine preoperative screening laboratory testing is indicated although numerous tests may be recommended, as mentioned below.

Laboratory Tests

Hemoglobin determination has been a standard preoperative test in many institutions. The discovery of anemia before hysterectomy may lead to cancellation of the surgery or prevent the need for transfusion and is therefore justified.

Urinalysis is another important preoperative indicator for potential morbidity, especially when the hysterectomy is associated with a urologic procedure. A complete urinalysis therefore is recommended with appropriate follow-up and pre- or intraoperative treatment.

A blood sample for typing and screening for unusual antibodies is usually sent to the blood bank prior to every hysterectomy.

A creatinine or blood urea nitrogen determination should be ordered in all women with a history of renal disease and those on antibiotics with primarily renal excretion. If all patients are screened, the incidence of abnormal values is 2.5% under age 40, 5% between ages 40 and 59 and 7.5% over age 60. Some physicians therefore believe that testing should be done in all women over age 60.

Determination of electrolyte levels is indicated in patients on diuretics or with a history of water or electrolyte imbalance.

Another important test to be considered is the blood glucose level in the morbidly obese, as well as in women with a history of diabetes. Liver function tests are indicated only if there is a history of liver disease.

Chest Radiograph

Routine preoperative chest radiographs have been seriously questioned in the literature. However, many textbooks still state, "chest x-ray examination is a routine hospital admission procedure."[4] In Rucker et al's review of 905 surgical patients, 386 were without risk factors and only one (0.3%) had an abnormal film.[8] They recommended chest radiographs in patients over the age of 60, and in patients with cardiopulmonary complaints or disease. Umbach et al found on a gynecologic service that only 1 of 1,175 patients would have received inappropriate treatment without chest radiography.[9] They recommended using chest radiographs only in patients with suspected pelvic malignancy and patients with cardiopulmonary disease.

Electrocardiogram

The general consensus about preoperative electrocardiography appears to be that an electrocardiogram (ECG) should be obtained in patients over the age of 40 and patients with cardiovascular complaints or disease.[10] McCleane studied 877 patients and found 45% to have abnormal ECGs.[11] The highest incidence appeared in patients over 40 and in patients of American Society of Anesthesiology grades II, III, IV, and V. They therefore recommended ECGs in these patients.

Systems Evaluations for Risk Factors

Respiratory System

An evaluation of the respiratory system is needed to identify those patients who are at high risk to develop pulmonary complications intra- and postoperatively. In approximately 10% of gynecologic operations, the postoperative course is complicated by atelectasis. This is more common in abdominal than in vaginal hysterectomies.

The history should include specific questions about dyspnea, sputum production, cough, wheezing, and past pulmonary problems, including smoking. If there is a history of pulmonary disease, a detailed medication history is very important. Any patient with a history of inhalation or oral corticosteroid use during the past 9 months should receive a parenteral corticosteroid to cover adrenal insufficiency. During the physical examination, special attention needs to be given to wheezing, rhonchi, rales, and tachypnea, as well as thorax movement. There should at least a 10-day interval between an upper respiratory infection and elective surgery.

All patients with positive findings on physical examination, as well as every patient with pulmonary disease, should have a chest radiograph and pulmonary function tests. Pulmonary function tests (spirometry) measure lung volumes and flow rates to help distinguish restrictive from obstructive pulmonary disease. The two most commonly used values are the vital capacity and the forced expiratory volume in 1 second (FEV_1). The vital capacity should be greater than 50% of predicted normal and the FEV_1 more than 75%. Stein and coworkers related the incidence of postoperative morbidity to preoperative pulmonary evaluation results. Among 33 patients with normal screening pulmonary function studies, there was one pulmonary complication, whereas among 30 with abnormal studies, there were 21 complications (70%).[12] However, Lawrence et al, in a review of 22 clinical articles about the predictive value of preoperative spirometry, found that spirometry's predictive value is unproven. Patients with moderate or severe lung disease also need an arterial blood gas measurement.[13] A large decrease in PaO_2 or a significant increase in $PaCO_2$ are especially indicative of severe problems during surgery, as well as in the postoperative period.

Other factors that contribute significantly to the rate of postoperative pulmonary complications include smoking, obesity, age, abdominal surgery, and pulmonary disease. It is therefore imperative to address these issues preoperatively with all patients.

Smoking is a significant factor in producing respiratory symptoms and in the development of obstructive lung disease. Physiologic changes that have been reported in smokers include increased airway resistance, decreased flow rates, decrease in surfactant activity, and decrease in basic lung defense mechanism through decreased macrophage activity. Smokers have a fourfold risk of pulmonary complications. Patients are advised to abstain from smoking for 2 to 4 weeks before their operation; however, even 12 to 72 hours of abstinence normalizes several important parameters.[14]

Obesity is another important risk factor. A body weight more than 20% above the ideal can double the pulmonary complications because the functional residual capacity is significantly reduced.[15]

With age there are changes in air flow rates, lung volumes, and elasticity leading to less efficient respiratory function. The rate of postoperative respiratory complications rises sharply after age 50.

Abdominal hysterectomy increases the rate of postoperative lung complications, especially atelectasis. Several studies showed that the vital capacity after abdominal surgery decreased.[16] This could therefore play a role in the decision whether to perform a vaginal versus an abdominal hysterectomy, especially when the patient has one or more of the above-mentioned risk factors.

Restrictive pulmonary disease (eg, fibrosis, pulmonary edema, pleural disease, neuromuscular disease and obesity) is characterized by a reduction in lung volume. The vital capacity and the FEV_1 are reduced but the ratio is normal. Usually there is hypoxemia without hypercapnia, which can be corrected by giving oxygen. Preoperative preparation includes use of incentive spirometry, especially if hypercapnia is present.

Obstructive pulmonary disease (asthma, bronchitis, and emphysema) is characterized by decreased expiratory flow rates. The vital capacity is usually normal, but the FEV_1 is reduced. Although these diseases are closely related, it is important to understand the differences. Bronchial asthma is an episodic disease manifested by general narrowing of the airways. Preoperative preparation should include removal of all allergenic materials and treatment with bronchodilators, humidification, hydration, and antibiotics if indicated. Bronchitis is a chronic disease characterized by excessive mucus secretion in the bronchial tree. The patient with bronchitis is therefore optimally treated with bronchodilators, decongestants, expectorants, and mucolytics. Preoperative therapy should be theophylline based, and adrenergic agents should be added when bronchospasm is present, either orally or as an inhaler. Emphysema is an anatomic abnormality consisting of abnormal enlargement of the distal air spaces secondary to destructive changes in the alveolar walls. These patients have a permanent change in their lungs and treatment is therefore not very successful. All medications with respiratory depressant capacity (especially morphine and meperidine) need to be used with great care in the patient with obstructive lung disease. If hypercapnia is present, oxygen use should be carefully monitored, since the possibility of respiratory depression is present.

Data substantiate that prophylactic measures do decrease postoperative complications. Preoperative measures that are recommended include: patient education, stopping smoking, training in proper breathing, bronchodilation, control of infection, and weight reduction (if indicated).[16]

Cardiovascular System

Most women with well-controlled cardiovascular disease can tolerate planned hysterectomy without any problems. However, the physiologic responses to pain, volume loss, and surgery include an increase in catecholamines, which increases cardiac output, conserves water, and maintains perfusion of vital organs. This in turn causes an increase in myocardial oxygen demand. There are a few conditions for which this is potentially very dangerous. These include congestive heart failure, a recent myocardial infarct, severe coronary artery disease, and poorly controlled hypertension.[17]

Nine cardiac risk factors were identified by Goldman et al in 1977.[18] These are age greater than 70, prior myocardial infarction within the preceding 6 months, presence of a third heart sound or jugular venous distention, important valvular aortic stenosis, rhythm other than sinus or premature atrial contractions, more than five premature ventricular contractions per minute prior to surgery, emergency operation, poor general medical condition, and intraperitoneal, intrathoracic, or aortic operation.

A good history will easily identify patients with cardiovascular problems. Questions should address exercise tolerance, shortness of breath, chest pain, edema, orthopnea, and previous cardiovascular history, including medications. On physical examination, blood pressure, abnormal heart rate or rhythm, murmur, pulmonary rales, and other signs of heart failure should be noted. A chest radiograph and resting as well as exercise ECG or nuclear scans should be ordered as indicated. For most gynecologists this will be done through a cardiology consultant.

Coronary Artery Disease

Coronary artery disease is mostly encountered in the postmenopausal woman, especially one with diabetes, hyperlipidemia, hypertension, or obesity. Unstable angina is a strong contraindication to surgery. Before elective hysterectomy, the patient should undergo a cardiac catheterization and stabilization of her disease. If the hysterectomy is emergent (eg, for bleeding), invasive hemodynamic monitoring should be performed intra- and postoperatively. When the patient has had a myocardial infarction, it is imperative to delay the surgery at least 6 months. This reduces mortality from around 30% at 3 months to 5% after 6 months.[19] Finally, it must be remembered that most postoperative myocardial infarctions occur in the first 3 to 4 days, and 60% of these present without chest pain.[20] The patient with coronary artery disease therefore must be monitored very closely during this period.

Congestive heart failure is one of the most important predictors of cardiac complications. It is therefore imperative to screen a patient well for any signs or symptoms of this disease and aggressively treat it prior to surgery. If emergency surgery is required, invasive monitoring is needed.

Valvular Heart Disease

Significant aortic stenosis has been associated with a mortality rate of up to 13% after noncardiac surgery and appears to be an independent risk factor.[21] However, this abnormality is fairly uncommon in the gynecologic population. The most common abnormality that the gynecologist will encounter is the mitral valve prolapse, which affects about 6% to 8% of women and is usually asymptomatic. Only those women with associated insufficiency need antibiotic prophylaxis, as well as those women with replacement valves, congenital anomalies, or other valvular disease.[22] The current antibiotic regimen before hysterectomy includes ampicillin 1 to 2 g intravenously (IV) and gentamycin 1.5 mg/kg prior to surgery. The dose needs to be repeated 6 to 8 hours later for maximal protection. For penicillin allergy, 1 g vancomycin can be substituted.

For women on anticoagulation therapy, studies show that the oral anticoagulants can be stopped safely 2 to 3 days prior to surgery. The patient is then admitted for heparin anticoagulation 2 days prior to surgery. If on admission the ratio of prothrombin time to normal clotting time is greater than 1.2, fresh frozen plasma or vitamin K can be given. The heparin is stopped 6 hours prior to surgery and restarted as soon as possible after surgery (usually 6 hours). Coumadin therapy is restarted immediately when oral intake is resumed.

Hypertension

When blood pressure is stable and the diastolic pressure is less than 110 mm Hg, no benefit is derived from postponing elective surgery.[23] If a woman has unstable hypertension or a diastolic pressure over 115 mm

Hg, especially in the presence of cardiac or renal disease, intensive preoperative medical treatment is indicated. Antihypertensive medication should be continued until the time of surgery and can usually be reinstituted when the patient resumes oral intake.

The most common perioperative hypertensive episodes are at the time of intubation (17% of women with hypertension), within the first hours after surgery, and approximately 48 hours after surgery.[24] Diuretics can lead to hypokalemia with its associated arrhythmias, and this must be corrected prior to surgery. A withdrawal syndrome can occur 24 to 48 hours after discontinuation of β-blockers, so these should be continued perioperatively. Clonidine can produce a rebound hypertension, and intravenous nitroprusside may be indicated. Transdermal clonidine can be instituted 48 to 72 hours prior to surgery. For the angiotensin-converting enzyme inhibitors and calcium channel blockers, intravenous substitution includes intravenous nitroprusside or hydralazine. However, intravenous substitution is only indicated for hypertension.

Thromboembolism

Postoperative thrombophlebitis and pulmonary embolism are among the most serious complications of hysterectomy. The incidence for leg vein thromboses in low-risk patients is less than 3%, whereas in high-risk patients (previous thromboembolism, hysterectomies for malignant disease, morbid obesity, and immobilization) it ranges from 30% to 60%.[24] The level of risk should be determined during the preoperative evaluation. Risk factors include history of previous thromboembolism, malignancy, immobilization, venous disease, use of oral contraceptives up to the time of hysterectomy, and lengthy operative procedure.

Oral contraceptives should be stopped 4 weeks prior to elective hysterectomies. Postmenopausal estrogen therapy can be continued until surgery. If patients fall in the high-risk category, preoperative subcutaneous heparin prophylaxis is started 2 hours prior to surgery and continued every 12 hours until full mobilization is reached. For long procedures, intraoperative pneumatic inflated sleeve devices on both legs may be used. These can also be used postoperatively but tend to decrease early mobilization. In several studies no difference in wound hematoma or postoperative bleeding was found with the use of mini-dose heparin. However, there are some women completely anticoagulated with this dose of heparin.

Gastrointestinal Tract

During history taking, gastrointestinal symptoms may be noted in the patient presenting for hysterectomy. These may be a change in stools, pain or bleeding with defecation, or blood or a mass detected on rectal examination. The appropriate consultation should be obtained, and these patients usually undergo radiologic studies as well as an endoscopic examination. It used to be routine to order a barium enema for every patient with an adnexal mass, but in this era of cost containment this no longer seems indicated. We do recommend barium enema for older patients with a left-sided adnexal mass and bowel symptoms.

It is no longer routine to admit patients the night before surgery for bowel cleansing. Some gynecologists believe that, for an elective hysterectomy where no cancer or adhesions are expected, there is no need for bowel preparation other than no oral intake for at least 6 hours prior to surgery. Some physicians give an enema the night before a hysterectomy to decrease contamination of the operative field and obtain a proper large bowel cleansing.

If there is suspicion that the operation may involve entry into the bowel, as in cases of severe endometriosis, adhesions, or an anticipated ovarian cancer, a complete bowel cleansing is indicated, including mechanical as well as antibiotic preparation. Studies of the techniques are abundant in the colorectal literature. A review of the most recent literature reveals that, if the patient is in good health, a home regimen is well tolerated.[25,26] The older 3-day regimen is therefore not used as much, especially by younger surgeons.[27,28] Current recommendations include clear liquids the day before surgery and administration of an oral gut lavage solution (Golytely) at a rate of 1.5 L/h for a total of 4 L or until the diarrhea is clear. No electrolyte disturbances have been found.[25] Occasionally a patient is unable to tolerate the solution and a nasogastric tube must be placed. Some surgeons advocate the use of tap water enemas on the day of surgery until the effluent is clear. On the same day, oral antibiotics are given. Different regimens have been used; most contain neomycin (1 g orally [PO]) given 3 to 4 times and erythromycin base (1 g PO) or Flagyl 3 to 4 times. Intravenous antibiotics are given right before surgery. If patients are aged or malnourished, or have medical problems, our policy is to admit them the day prior to surgery to prevent dehydration.

Urinary Tract

Gynecologic disease may produce anatomic disturbance of the urinary tract. It used to be standard practice to order an intravenous pyelogram (IVP) to determine urinary tract anatomy before every major gynecologic procedure. In the last 5 years, however, several studies have addressed the use of IVP in these cases. There are no studies that prove that a preoperative IVP prevents ureteral injury. The estimated incidence of ureteral injury is 0.5% to 2.5% for all gynecologic operations.[29,30] The congenital anomalies found with IVP are important but rare (1% to 6%).[31] Approximately 5% to 8% of women will have an allergic reaction to IVP dye, with 1% to 2% of these reactions being very serious.

Piscitelli et al reviewed 493 cases in 1987 and found that, of the 60.6% of patients who underwent an IVP prior to hysterectomy, 27% had an abnormal test.[29] The clinical factors likely to be associated with an abnormal IVP included uterine size greater than the equivalent of 12 weeks of pregnancy or an adnexal mass larger than 4 cm. Not associated with an abnormal IVP were endometriosis, previous abdominal surgery, pelvic inflammatory disease, or pelvic relaxation, although in their discussion the authors stated that their sample size may not have been big enough to detect such associations. The abnormalities found included 6% congenital anomalies, 10.6% ureteral dilation, and 4.7% ureteral dilation. In this group two ureteral injuries were found at the time of vaginal hysterectomy, one in each group (IVP and no IVP). To answer the question of whether preoperative IVP decreases the incidence of ureteral injury, a study with 11,450 patients is needed, which would cost over $5 million. According to the available data, the decision to perform a preoperative IVP should be based on an abnormal clinical and physical examination, with the knowledge that the only way to prevent a ureteral injury is to extensively evaluate the location of the ureter intraoperatively.

Insufficient renal function is a major risk factor in elective operations. Therefore, as outlined before, a good history and physical examination, as well as kidney function studies when indicated, are of the utmost importance.

Preoperative, Prophylactic Antibiotic Usage

Prophylactic antibiotic therapy refers to antibiotics given before surgery in a way that will ensure a tissue level of medication before the operation occurs. This has been shown clearly to reduce postoperative febrile morbidity in premenopausal patients undergoing vaginal hysterectomy. It has been of less obvious benefit in postmenopausal patients undergoing vaginal hysterectomy, or in patients of any age who are undergoing abdominal hysterectomy. Patients who have selected factors that reduce their own immune system competence or that increase infection risks may benefit from antibiotic prophylaxis regardless of the method of hysterectomy used, or the age of the patient at surgery. These factors would include patients with morbid obesity, bacterial vaginosis, previous pelvic infections, ongoing immunosuppressing illnesses or medications, or other evidence for natural interference with host defense mechanisms.

Adjunctive techniques to prevent postoperative febrile morbidity, and especially wound infections, have been extensively evaluated by Cruse and Ford.[32] Shaving of pubic hair on the night before surgery is no longer recommended; instead, hair is clipped at the time of surgery. Likewise, vaginal douching the night before surgery has been shown to be less effective than thorough cleansing of the vagina with a povidone-iodine solution immediately prior to surgery in the operating room. A shower with antiseptic soap on the evening before surgery remains a helpful adjunct to infection prevention. Scheduling surgery in the preovulatory phase of the menstrual cycle may also reduce postoperative morbidity.

Many different regimens have been recommended for prophylactic antibiotic therapy for hysterectomy. Holman and coworkers described a perioperative regimen using cefazolin, a broad-spectrum cephalosporin.[33] Hemsell et al have shown that 1 g of cefazolin given IV or intramuscularly before surgery as a single dose is effective in preventing postoperative infections.[34] Orr and associates have even shown a reduction in febrile morbidity in patients undergoing abdominal hysterectomy with the use of a single preoperative 2-g dose of cefotetan, another long-acting, broad-spectrum cephalosporin with β-lactamase stability.[35]

Certainly standards for subacute bacterial endocarditis prevention (SBE prophylaxis) should be maintained for patients undergoing hysterectomy. Usually ampicillin 1.5 g IV with gentamycin 80 mg IV, given 30 to 60 minutes preoperatively, is sufficient for patients with abnormal cardiac blood flow, including valvular heart disease (with mitral valve prolapse being most common). For persons with penicillin allergies, vancomycin 1.0 g IV given *slowly* 1 hour prior to surgery, or clindamycin 600 mg IV and gentamicin 80 mg IV given 30 to 60 minutes preoperatively, is also effective.

References

1. Rosoff AJ: *Informed Consent: A Guide for Health Care Providers.* London, Aspen Publ, 1981, p 1.
2. *Schloendorff v Society of New York Hospital*, 211 NY 125, 105 N.E. 92, 93 (1914).
3. American College of Obstetricians and Gynecologists Committee on Ethics: *Ethical Dimensions of Informed Consent.* Committee Opinion No. 108. Washington, DC, American College of Obstetricians and Gynecologists, 1992.
4. Freeman MG: Psychological aspects of pelvic surgery, in Thomson JD, Rock JA (eds): *TeLinde's Operative Gynecology*, ed 7. Philadelphia, JB Lippincott Co, 1992, pp 13–22.
5. Roeske NCA: Hysterectomy and other gynecologic surgery: A psychological view, in Notman MT, Nadelson CC (eds): *The Woman Patient: Medical and Psychological Interfaces.* New York, Plenum Press, 1978.
6. Kaplan EB, Scheiner LB, Boeckmann AJ, et al: The usefulness of preoperative laboratory screening. *JAMA* 1985;253:3576–3581.
7. Narr BJ, Hansen TR, Warner MA: Preoperative laboratory screening in healthy Mayo patients: Cost effective elimination of test and unchanged outcomes. *Mayo Clin Proc* 1991;66:155–159.
8. Rucker L, Frye EB, Staten MA: Usefulness of screening chest roentgenograms in preoperative patients. *JAMA* 1983;250:3209–3211.
9. Umbach GE, Zubeck S, Deck HJ, et al: The value of preoperative chest x-rays in gynecological patients. *Arch Gynecol Obstet* 1988;243:179–186.
10. Goldberger AL, O'Konski M: Utility of the routine electrocardiogram before surgery and on general hospital.
11. McCleane GJ, McCoy E: Routine preoperative electro-cardiography. *Br J Clin Pract* 1990;44:92–95.

12. Stein M, Koota GM, Simon M, et al: Pulmonary evaluation of surgical patients. *JAMA* 1962;181:765–770.
13. Lawrence VA, Page CP, Harris GD: Preoperative spirometry before abdominal operations. A critical appraisal of its predictive value. *Arch Intern Med* 1989;149:280–285.
14. Anderson ME, Belani KG: Short-term preoperative smoking abstinence. *Am Fam Physician* 1990;41:1191–1194.
15. Wiren JE, Janzon L: Respiratory complications following surgery. Improved prediction with preoperative spirometry. *Acta Anaesthesiol Scand* 1983;27:47–49.
16. Tisi GM: Preoperative identification and evaluation of the patient with lung disease. *Med Clin North Am* 1987;71:399–412.
17. Weitz HH, Goldman L: Noncardiac surgery in the patient with heart disease. *Med Clin North Am* 1987;71:413–432.
18. Goldman L, Caldera DL, Nussbaum SR, et al: Multi-factorial index of cardiac risk in noncardiac surgical procedures. *N Engl J Med* 1977;297:845–850.
19. DeBusk R, Blomquist C, Kouchoukos N, et al: Identification and treatment of low risk patients after acute myocardial infarction and coronary artery bypass after surgery. *N Engl J Med* 1986;314:161–166.
20. Sten P, Tinker J, Tarhan S: Myocardial reinfarction after anesthesia and surgery. *JAMA* 1978;239:2566–2570.
21. Goldman L, Caldera D, Southwick F, et al: Cardiac risk factors and complications in non-cardiac surgery. *Medicine* 1978;57:357–370.
22. Shulman S, Amren DP, Bisno AL, et al: Prevention of bacterial endocarditis. *Circulation* 1984;70:1123A–1127A.
23. Goldman L, Caldera D: Risks of general anesthesia and elective operation in the hypertensive patient. *Anesthesiology* 1979;50:285–292.
24. Bonnar T: Venous thrombo embolism and gynecologic surgery. *Clin Obstet Gynecol* 1984;28:435–446.
25. Beck DE, Fazio VW: Current preoperative bowel cleansing methods. Results of a survey. *Dis Colon Rectum* 1990;33:12–15.
26. Frazee RC, Robert J, Symmonds R, et al: Prospective, randomized trial of inpatient vs outpatient bowel preparation for elective colorectal surgery. *Dis Colon Rectum* 1992;35:233–236.
27. Huddy SP, Rayter Z, Webber PP, et al: Preparation of the bowel before elective surgery using a polyethylene glycol solution at home and in hospital compared with conventional preparation using magnesium sulphate. *J R Coll Surg Edinb* 1990;35:16–20.
28. Beck DE, Manford FJ, diPalma JA: Comparison of cleansing methods in preparation for colonic surgery. *Dis Colon Rectum* 1985;28:491–495.
29. Piscitelle JT, Simel DL, Addison WA: Who should have intravenous pyelograms before hysterectomy for benign disease? *Obstet Gynecol* 1987;69:541–545.
30. Sack RA: The value of intravenous urography prior to abdominal hysterectomy for gynecological disease. *Am J Obstet Gynecol* 1979;134:208–212.
31. Klissaristose AA, Manouelides NS, Comninos AC: Preoperative intravenous pyelography in gynecology. *Int Surg* 1974;59:31–32.
32. Cruse PJE, Foord R: The epidemiology of wound infection: A 10 year prospective study of 939 wounds. *Surg Clin North Am* 1980;60:27–48.

33. Holman JF, McGowan JE, Thompson JD: Perioperative antibiotics in major elective gynecologic surgery. *South Med J* 1978;71:417–420.
34. Hemsell DI, Reisch J, Nobles BJ, et al: Single dose prophylaxis for vaginal and abdominal hysterectomy. *Am J Obstet Gynecol* 1978;147:520–525.
35. Orr JR, Varner RE, Kilgore LC, et al: Cefotetan v. cefoxitin as prophylaxis in hysterectomy. *Am J Obstet Gynecol* 1986;154:960–964.

Chapter **2**

Current Indications for Hysterectomy

M. Chrystie Timmons, MD, and W. Allen Addison, MD

Hysterectomy is the second most commonly performed major operation in the United States, with a reported annual rate of 6.7 per 1,000 women and with more than 650,000 hysterectomies being performed per year[1-3] at an annual cost of $3 billion. Hysterectomy is second only to cesarean section in frequency of major operations in the United States. The mortality rate for either abdominal or vaginal hysterectomy is 1 to 2 per 1,000.[4]

Because of the frequency with which hysterectomy is performed, the annual health care costs arising from hysterectomy, and regional variations in justification of hysterectomy,[5] the indications for hysterectomy have attracted widespread attention. This attention has come from such diverse quarters as patient awareness and consumer groups, third-party payment providers (both government and private), and peer review and quality assurance processors. The indications for hysterectomy are multiple, ranging from indisputably life-threatening conditions such as uncontrollable obstetric hemorrhage, as might be seen with placenta accreta and the Couvelaire uterus, or uterine malignancy, to the usually non–life-threatening conditions of leiomyomata, endometriosis, and dysfunctional bleeding uncontrolled with medical management. An additional important category of indications is the varying degrees of prolapse that can best be managed by hysterectomy, which is technically elective but can relieve discomfort and improve a woman's quality of life enormously in a nonqualifiable manner.

Further confounding the difficulty in assessing valid indications for hysterectomy is the ongoing evolution of both medical and hormonal managements for such problems as dysmenorrhea and dysfunctional uterine bleeding. In like manner, over the years new surgical techniques have evolved that have provided therapeutic alternatives to hysterectomy in select patterns. For example, the use of danocrine, progesterones, and gonadotropin-releasing hormone (GnRH) agonists may effectively treat the symptomatology and pathology of endometriosis, thereby avoiding hysterectomy at a given point in time or indefinitely. Examples of surgical alternatives to hysterectomy include hysteroscopic resection of submucosal uterine leiomyomata, endometrial ablation for recalcitrant bleeding, and the series of techniques for treating cervical intraepithelial neoplasia (CIN) from cryotherapy through laser to loop electrosurgical excision of the transformation zone (LEETZ).

The purpose of this chapter is to consider contemporary opinions regarding indications for hysterectomy. An understanding of the history, the past and present epidemiology, and current alternatives to hysterectomy is essential for selecting those patients who will benefit from hysterectomy.

History of Hysterectomy

An excellent historical and current critical review of hysterectomy is provided by Bachman.[7] The first recorded hysterectomy occurred in Greece 17 centuries ago with removal of a gangrenous, inverted uterus. Because of a mortality rate of approximately 90%, hysterectomy was rarely performed until advances of anesthesia and aseptical surgical technique allowed reduction in the mortality rate. The first subtotal hysterectomy was performed by Heath in 1843 for an enlarged uterus. In 1850, Burnham performed the first total abdominal hysterectomy. Mortality rates for vaginal hysterectomy dropped from 15% in 1890 to 2.5% in 1910, and for abdominal hysterectomy from over 70% in 1880 to 3% by 1930.[8] With continuing improvements in anesthesia, the advent of antibiotics, and development of surgical instruments and techniques, the morbidity and mortality of hysterectomy has continued to decrease. These developments have more safely afforded the benefits of hysterectomy to increasing numbers of women, with resulting increase in occurrence to levels requiring scrutiny.

Epidemiology of Hysterectomy

The rate of hysterectomy increased from 6.1 per 1,000 women in 1965 to a high of 8.6 per 1,000 women in 1975. This rate plateaued in the late 1970s and early 1980s at approximately 7 per 1,000 women. The highest rate of hysterectomy is found in women in their 30s and 40s (11 and 15 per 1,000, respectively), and the lowest rate of 3 per 1,000 women is found in women under 30. A mean age of approximately 42.7 years and a median age of 40.9 years have remained consistent in data collected from 1965 to 1987.[3]

There are marked differences in hysterectomy rates from country to country and from region to region within the same country. For example, the hysterectomy rate in 1984 in New Zealand was 4.1 per 1,000 women,[10] as compared to a rate of approximately 7.0 per 1,000 women in the United

States.[3] Furthermore, the rates in New Zealand reported from different hospital boards varied from 1.5 to 7.1 per 1,000 women. In an analysis of hysterectomy rates in 35 hospital catchment areas of one Canadian province, Roos found a fivefold variation attributed principally to physician practice patterns.[11] The hysterectomy rates in Europe were compared by Van Keep et al, who noted a low rate of 5.8 per 1,000 in France and a high rate of 15.5 per 1,000 in Italy.[12]

In the United States, the highest hysterectomy rate, particularly in younger women,[3] has occurred consistently in the South. There, the rate has been 2.5 times higher than the rate in the Northeast, which has consistently exhibited the lowest rate.[13] Rates for black women have been higher than those for white women from the beginning of surveillance in 1970 until 1982.[13]

Although the rates of hysterectomy have decreased in the United States since the mid-1970s, the absolute numbers of hysterectomies have continued to and are expected to increase because of our aging population (ie, there will be an increase in the group with the highest hysterectomy rates).[4] With increasing pressure to contain health care costs, the indications for hysterectomy have come under increased scrutiny, and programs have been developed in an attempt to control the performance of questionably indicated hysterectomies and to define objective criteria to guide hysterectomy indications. For example, the requirement by many third-party payers for a confirming second opinion prior to elective hysterectomy is an attempt to reduce the number of questionably indicated hysterectomies. In a study of second opinions in the New York City area, 24.7% of the second opinions did not concur with the need for the proposed hysterectomy.[14] In this study, the majority of discordance resulted from the opinion that the patient did not have symptoms of severity sufficient to warrant surgery, or that further evaluation was warranted before resorting to surgery. Another study by Finkel and Finkel,[15] looking at cross-regional second opinions through a major insurance carrier, showed a discordance of 8.0% without statistically significant regional or urban/rural differences. Of interest, however, was the fact that 53% of women in the North Central region and 55.6% of women in the South proceeded to have a hysterectomy despite a discordant second opinion.

The quality assurance process has been invoked in evaluating indications for hysterectomy. Gambone and associates[16] devised a system requiring the surgeon to select one preoperative indication for hysterectomy. The hysterectomy specimens were not expected to show pathology in 34% of the listed indications, and the validation of the hysterectomy indication had to be indicated by defined standards in the surgeon's preoperative notes (eg, demonstrable stress urinary incontinence documented by urodynamic testing). With this system, 584 consecutive hysterectomies were evaluated, with 93% of the "pathology expected" indications "verified" by the pathology report and 98% of the "no pathology expected" indications "validated" by the preoperative notes. A similar quality assurance review by Rizvi et al[17] also judged 92% of 250 hysterectomies as being indicated.

In summary, although hysterectomy rates appear to have reached a plateau and may decline because of advances in nonsurgical management, the absolute number of hysterectomies will continue to increase according to projections by the U.S. Bureau of the Census to 783,000 in 1995 and 824,000 in 2005.[18] With the increased scrutiny regarding justification of hysterectomy, gynecologists must stay continually current with the accepted indications for hysterectomy.

Indications for Hysterectomy

The five most common indications for hysterectomy in the United States from 1965 to 1987 were leiomyomata (30% of the total), endometriosis (19%), prolapse (16%), cancer (10%), and endometrial hyperplasia (6%). The remaining 19% of hysterectomies were performed because of abnormal bleeding, disorders of menstruation, or disorders of the parametrium.[3] Other infrequent indications include obstetric emergencies such as intractable hemorrhage, hysterectomy associated with life-threatening pelvic infection, ruptured interstitial ectopic pregnancy, abortion, and sterilization.

Leiomyomata

Uterine leiomyomata have consistently been the leading indication for hysterectomy in the United States[1,3,4,7,15,16,19] and in other countries.[8,20–22] Most (83%) of the hysterectomies performed for the indication of leiomyomata are in the 35- to 54-year-old age group.[3] Pathology confirmation of this preoperative indication is high. In Gambone et al's report,[16] 88% of hysterectomies for leiomyomata were confirmed by pathology reports, and 96% were confirmed if criteria allowed alternatively acceptable pathology (eg, an adnexal mass considered to be contiguous with the uterus preoperatively). In a follow-up study, after the institution of a criteria-based quality assurance program, 94% (217/230) of the preoperative diagnoses of leiomyomata were confirmed by pathology reports.[23] Therefore, if the indication for hysterectomy is leiomyomata, pathology confirmation is expected. In general, leiomyomata as an indication for hysterectomy is for management of secondary symptoms, which might consist of abnormal bleeding, pelvic pain, or pelvic pressure. Although it is debated by some investigators, asymptomatic leiomyomata may constitute an indication for hysterectomy because of absolute size (equivalent to 12 to 14 weeks of pregnancy), which may make bimanual examination of the pelvis suboptimal. Rapid uterine enlargement exclusive of the possibility of leiomyosarcoma, and ureteral compression documented by intravenous pyelogram or renal-pelvic ultrasound, are widely accepted indications for hysterectomy.

Current available alternatives to hysterectomy for leiomyomata may have significant impact on the rate of such hysterectomies, the absolute number of which have increased by a total of over 100,000 for 1987 contrasted to the number of 1967.[3] Myomectomy, in spite of a significant recurrent rate of myomas,[24] is an alternative generally reserved for women who wish to retain childbearing potential and for women who will not accept hysterectomy in spite of uterine pathology and the likelihood of recurrent myomas. With the use of GnRH agonists, uterine volume is reduced by 20% to 60%,[7] with resultant decreased bleeding, but this benefit is temporary. Thus, pretreatment of the patient with GnRH agonist is generally viewed as a surgical adjuvant. However, it may also be suitable for the perimenopausal patient in whom leiomyomata can be expected to shrink following menopause. If the source of abnormal bleeding is secondary to a submucosal leiomyomata, hysteroscopic resection of the leiomyoma may successfully treat the symptom and underlying pathology without the need for hysterectomy.

Endometriosis

Endometriosis is the second most common indication for hysterectomy, with a sharply increasing rate between 1965 and 1987, surpassing genital prolapse and cancer in frequency of indication for hysterectomy in this 22-year interval.[3] Most (75%) of the hysterectomies for endometriosis are done in the 25- to 44-year-old age group, which is a younger group than those who undergo hysterectomy for leiomyomata. Hysterectomies for endometriosis now account for 19% of all hysterectomies performed.[4] The marked increase of 121%[4] from 1965 to 1987 may reflect an increased prevalence of the condition or improved ability to diagnose the condition with laparascopy.[7] It should be noted, however, that the increase in the rate of hysterectomy because of endometriosis actually was established in 1965, before laparoscopy was widely used. Endometriosis, like leiomyomata, has a high rate (88% to 92%) of confirmation by pathology report.[16,23]

With improved alternatives to hysterectomy for endometriosis over the last decade, the rate of hysterectomy for endometriosis may decline. For example, laparoscopy allows not only earlier diagnosis in a younger population, but treatment by resection, cautery, or laser[25] at an earlier stage of disease. Primary or adjunctive medical therapy with low-dose oral contraceptives, danazol, progesterones, or GnRH agonists may arrest or control endometriosis, thereby decreasing or eliminating the symptoms of chronic pelvic pain and dyspareunia. These therapies, however, are often expensive and may have undesirable side effects, and residual endometriosis may well reactivate after therapy is discontinued. For many women who do not desire to maintain their reproductive capacity, abdominal hysterectomy with bilateral salpingo-oophorectomy provides definitive surgical therapy and can be justified on a cost-effectiveness basis, if the cost of doctor visits, medication, and minor procedures are weighed, as well as on the basis of an improved quality of life.

Prolapse

Urogenital prolapse is the third most frequent indication for hysterectomy, accounting for 16% of all hysterectomies in the United States.[3] This is the most frequent indication for hysterectomy in women 65 years old and older, surpassing cancer as an indication.[13] Histologically confirmed pathology is not expected in this group, but verification and documentation in the preoperative surgeon's notes has been shown to be as high as 100%.[16] This indication for hysterectomy also includes hysterectomies performed in conjunction with procedures for treatment of stress urinary incontinence. Of vaginal hysterectomies performed, 39% have a preoperative diagnosis of vaginal relaxation or uterine descensus listed.[26]

The alternatives to hysterectomy for significant prolapse are of limited value. Once symptomatic uterine prolapse with accompanying anterior and/or posterior vaginal wall relaxation through the introitus has occurred, surgical correction is usually indicated.[27] Kegel exercises alone or enhanced by biofeedback may provide enough improvement in symptomatology that hysterectomy with adjunctive reconstructive operations for relaxation may not be necessary as long as the progress of the prolapse is arrested and exercises are continued. Pessary use may also be of some value in patients who are poor operative candidates or who do not desire surgical correction. Reconstructive surgery for urogenital prolapse is aimed at improving the patient's quality of life.

Cancer

Cancer was the indication for 10% of hysterectomies from 1965 to 1987 in the United States.[3] This accounted for 33% of the indications for hysterectomies in women 65 years of age and older versus only 7.8% in the other age groups combined.[3] This indication has a high correlation (100%) with pathology evaluations.[23] Conservation of the uterus in uterine and/or ovarian cancer must be individualized according to the patient's age, desire for future childbearing, and specific malignant pathology.

Endometrial Hyperplasia

Endometrial hyperplasia accounts for 6% of hysterectomies[3] and also has a high (100%) correlation with the pathology report.[23] The rationale for hysterectomy for endometrial hyperplasia is based on the concept that endometrial hyperplasia is a premalignant condition and has the potential to progress to actual uterine cancer. Most gynecologists agree that a trial of progesterone therapy, endometrial sampling, and dilation and curettage are the therapeutic modalities of choice before considering hysterectomy for endometrial hyperplasia without associated atypia. In the face of significant atypia, hyperplasia in a postmenopausal woman receiving no exogenous estrogen, or persistent hyperplasia despite progesterone therapy, hysterectomy is considered by most to be the treatment of choice.

Other Indications

Approximately 20% of hysterectomies are performed for a variety of other reasons: abnormal bleeding without obvious cause, obstetric emergencies (uterine rupture, placenta previa/accreta, abruption with Couvelaire uterus, ruptured cornual ectopic), pelvic arteriovenous malformation, infection, adnexal pathology, abortion and sterilization, and "elective."[3] Likewise, intraoperative attempts to control uterine hemorrhage of obstetric etiology by means of drug therapy (pitocin, prostaglandins), mechanical means (uterine packing), or alternative surgical approaches (uterine artery ligation, bilateral hypogastric artery ligation) are worthwhile as long as these attempts are not prolonged in an unstable patient with life-threatening hemorrhage.

Although there have been proponents for hysterectomy to accomplish sterilization[28,29] and sterilization-abortion,[30] this is difficult to justify when related to the increased risk, pain, and expense as compared to other methods of sterilization.[31,32] One subset of patients in whom hysterectomy for sterilization may be applicable is profoundly retarded patients in whom the problem of menstrual hygiene as well as sterilization can be addressed by hysterectomy.

Purely elective hysterectomy in a patient without gynecologic symptoms or pathology, or in most patients as a prophylaxis against cancer, can usually be justified, although extenuating circumstances such as patient anxiety or phobia may exist.[7]

Conclusions

There are many appropriate indications for hysterectomy, and there are hysterectomies performed without good indications. Good indications for hysterectomy can be considered in three broad categories: to save a life, to correct pathology that interferes with function, and to improve the quality of life.[7] It behooves the gynecologic surgeon, in the current atmosphere of increased scrutiny and justification of hysterectomy indications, to keep meticulous medical records, provide careful preoperative notes, and use appropriate preoperative diagnostic tests. Patients need to be well informed regarding the preoperative diagnosis, proposed surgical plan, and anticipated benefits and risks of alternative medical or surgical therapies. Although the mortality of hysterectomy is low—1 to 2 per 1,000 hysterectomies (pooled data of all types, all indications)—significant numbers of women undergoing hysterectomy will experience some perioperative complication or morbidity. The gynecologist must therefore evaluate the risks (morbidity, mortality, surgical goal not accomplished) and benefits (saving of life, improved quality of life) for each patient in terms of the indication for hysterectomy.

References

1. National Center for Health Statistics: 1982 summary. National hospital discharge survey (No. 95). *Vital Health Stat* 1983.
2. Easterday CL, Grimes DA, Riggs JA: Hysterectomy in the United States. *Obstet Gynecol* 1983;62:203–212.
3. Pokras R: Hysterectomy: Past, present, and future. *Stat Bull Metrop Insur Co* 1989;70:12.
4. Pokras R, Hufnagel VG: Hysterectomies in the United States, 1965–84. *Am J Public Health* 1988;78:852–853.
5. Wingo PA, Huezo CM, Rubin GL, et al: The mortality risk associated with hysterectomy. *Am J Obstet Gynecol* 1985;152:803–808.
6. Doyle JC: Unnecessary hysterectomies. *JAMA* 1953;151:360–365.
7. Bachman GA: Hysterectomy a critical review. *J Reprod Med* 1990;35:839–862.
8. Leonardo RA: *History of Gynecology*. New York, Froben Press, 1944.
9. Benrubi GI: History of hysterectomy. *J Fla Med Assoc* 1988;75:533–538.
10. Macintosh MC: Incidence of hysterectomy in New Zealand. *NZ Med J* 1987;100:345–347.
11. Roos NP: Hysterectomy: Variations in rates across small areas and across physicians' practices. *Am J Public Health* 1984;74:327.
12. van Keep PA, Wildemeersh D, Lehert P: Hysterectomy in six European countries. *Maturitas* 1983;5:69–75.
13. Irwin KL, Peterson HB, Hughes JM, et al: *MMWR CDC Surveill Summ* 1986;35:1SS.
14. McCarthy EG, Finkel ML: Second consultants opinion for elective gynecologic surgery. *Obstet Gynecol* 1980;56:403–410.
15. Finkel ML, Finkel DJ: The effect of a second opinion program on hysterectomy performance. *Med Care* 1990;28:776–783.
16. Gambone JC, Lench JB, Slasinski MJ, et al: Validation of hysterectomy indications and the quality assurance process. *Obstet Gynecol* 1989;73:1045–1049.
17. Rizvi JH, Afzal W, Ali A, et al: Was that hysterectomy really necessary? Audit of the operative justification at the Aga Khan University Medical Center, Karachi. *Aust N Z J Obstet Gynaecol* 1991;31:80–83.
18. US Bureau of the Census: Projection of the population of the United States, by age, sex, and race: 1983 to 2080, Current Population Reports Series P-25. Washington, DC, US Government Printing Office, 1984.
19. Amirikia H, Evans TN: Ten-year review of hysterectomies: Trends, indications, and risks. *Am J Obstet Gynecol* 1979;134:431–437.

20. Ramsewak S, Perkins S, Roopnarinesingh S: Indications and risks of abdominal hysterectomy. *W V Med J* 1988;37:215–217.
21. Loizzi P, Carriero C, DiGesu A, et al: Removal or preservation of ovaries during hysterectomy: A six year review. *Int J Gynecol Obstet* 1990;31:257–261.
22. Browne DS, Frazer MI: Hysterectomy revisited. *Aust N Z J Obstet Gynaecol* 1991;31:148–152.
23. Gambone JC, Reiter RC, Lench JB, et al: The impact of a quality assurance program on the frequency and confirmation rate of hysterectomy. *Am J Obstet Gynecol* 1990;163:545–550.
24. Malone LJ: Myomectomy: Recurrence after removal of solitary and multiple myomas. *Obstet Gynecol* 1969;34:200–203.
25. Keye WR Jr, Dixon J: Photocoagulation of endometriosis by the argon laser through the laparoscope. *Obstet Gynecol* 1983;62:383–386.
26. Copenhaver EH: Vaginal hysterectomy. An analysis of indications and complications among 1000 operations. *Am J Obstet Gynecol* 1962;84:123–127.
27. Mishell DR (ed): *Menopause: Physiology and Pharmacology.* Chicago, Year Book Medical Publishers, 1988.
28. Atkinson SM Jr, Chapell SM: Vaginal hysterectomy for sterilization. *Obstet Gynecol* 1972;39:759–766.
29. Grody MHT: Is vaginal hysterectomy justified as a method for sterilization? *J Gynecol Surg* 1989;5:313–315.
30. Stumpf PG, Ballard CA, Lowensohn R: Abdominal hysterectomy for abortion-sterilization. *Am J Obstet Gynecol* 1980;136:714–720.
31. Laros RK Jr, Work BA: Female sterilization: III. Vaginal hysterectomy. *Am J Obstet Gynecol* 1975;122:693–697.
32. Nichols DH: Is vaginal hysterectomy justified as a method for sterilization? *J Gynecol Surg* 1989;5:317–318.

Chapter **3**

Vaginal Versus Abdominal Hysterectomy

David H. Nichols, MD

About 650,000 hysterectomies are performed annually in the United States, and about 70% are done transabdominally and 30% transvaginally. The National Center for Health Statistics has determined that, as the number of women in the population increases in the coming years, so will the number of hysterectomies being done. Without changes in the hysterectomy rate, the prediction is that the number will rise to about 810,000 in 1995 and 854,000 in the year 2005.

There must be consideration of the true indications for hysterectomy in each particular patient, so that both the patient and surgeon can understand the reasons for the recommendations. Is the diagnosis clear cut? Is the patient anxious to be sterilized? Is surgery being recommended for the relief of some undiagnosed and ill-defined pelvic pain? Precision in diagnosis will be followed by precision in therapy and vast improvement in the operative results.

Choice of Surgical Approach

A hysterectomy can be accomplished either transvaginally or transabdominally. Provided the operating surgeon is competent in the techniques for both, the patient undergoing vaginal hysterectomy will generally have a more comfortable postoperative course. Unless an anterior or posterior colporraphy was done, a significantly shorter period of postoperative hospitalization is required, making the procedure more cost effective in a health care system in which the expense of hospitalization has never been higher, with every expectation that it will continue to rise in the years ahead. With vaginal hysterectomy, operating time is shorter, and there is no abdominal incision to make and close; therefore, bowel obstruction is infrequent, there are no wound hernias or wound infections, and there is no cosmetically unattractive scar on the abdomen. Because there is less bowel manipulation, there is significant reduction of postoperative ileus in the vaginal hysterectomy patient. The period of operative anesthesia is shorter, generally less than 2 hours, permitting the use of spinal anesthesia when desired, and because profound muscular relaxation is not required, the depth of anesthesia may be less when the operation is done transvaginally.

There are occasional champions of reintroduction of subtotal hysterectomy in the surgeon's choice of operation, citing alleged enhancement of coital response and pleasure. The subtotal, or cervix-sparing, operation can be performed through either a transabdominal or transvaginal approach, should this be an operative consideration or requirement. Similarly, myomectomy (or multiple myomectomy) as a surgical alternative can be planned through either exposure or approach depending on the operator's skill and experience.

The route chosen for hysterectomy should always be that which is in the best interests of the particular patient. Since the choice includes considerations pertaining to length of postoperative stay as well as the cost of operating time, the procedure should be affordable and at the same time cost effective. The surgeon should know and be experienced in the various routes of hysterectomy and thus choose that which best fits the needs and interests of a particular patient. The surgeon should avoid the temptation to employ only a single route with which he or she is most comfortable. As Lee has observed, the more we do of a procedure the better we get at it. However, choosing among three procedures performed frequently gives better results than choosing among 20 performed infrequently.

For most patients, hysterectomy can be safely accomplished by the transvaginal route, taking advantage of the cost-effective opportunity for a shorter duration of surgery, shorter hospitalization, and improved postoperative patient comfort. With each decision must come the opportunity to surgically correct any additional sites of anatomic damage and lessen the chance for recurrence of any deficiency of support. To the enthusiast the only indications for abdominal hysterectomy are the contraindications to vaginal hysterectomy! These contraindications are quite specific:

1. Lack of mobility of the uterus
2. Uterine size greater than the equivalent of 12 weeks' gestation
3. Presence of an adnexal tumor in which malignancy is a distinct possibility
4. Massively contracted bony pelvis
5. A clearcut need for exploring the remainder of the abdomen
6. Lack of surgeon experience and enthusiasm for the vaginal approach

Previous surgery, even cesarean section, is not a contraindication to vaginal hysterectomy. When there is a history of cesarean section, the patient's bladder should be emptied at the beginning of the operation, and 60 mL of dilute indigo carmine solution instilled. Since this solution stains the vesical mucosa, any violet discoloration of the tissue being dissected can be recognized instantly before cystotomy and the direction of dissection altered safely to a deeper layer.

Patient Education and Informed Consent

The patient should be a participant in the decision-making process and given a truly informed consent that will explain the various options for choice of route for hysterectomy, the therapeutic alternatives to hysterectomy, and the surgeon's recommendations for this particular patient, with a good explanation of why that specific recommendation has been made.

After the patient has been carefully examined and a decision made that hysterectomy is in her best interests, a thorough explanation of the various routes for hysterectomy and the alternatives to hysterectomy should be given thoughtfully and with abundant opportunity for the patient to pose any questions and discuss any details. She should be made aware of the usual convalescence, and given an opportunity to formulate and express her own ideas as to what surgery is to be done. It is valuable for the surgeon to know how the patient perceives her disease and its proposed remedy, and the effect it is likely to have on her future lifestyle and relationships.

Goals of Hysterectomy

The goals of hysterectomy, whether transvaginal or transabdominal, are (1) relief of symptoms, (2) restoration of normal anatomic relationships, and (3) restoration of function. The operation chosen for a particular patient should make it possible for these goals to be achieved. It is the second goal, restoration of normal anatomic relationships, that may result in confusion for the surgeon. Standard anatomic texts describe in detail the anatomic and organ relationships of the cadaver, but this is generally in sharp contrast to those of the living patient, in whom voluntary muscle tone and a normally empty rectum permit the vagina to lie on an intact levator plate. The upper vaginal axis is thus horizontal, and not vertical as is shown in description of cadaver anatomy. Restoration, support, and suspension of the vaginal vault into the hollow of the sacrum and over an intact levator plate is a major goal of reconstruction if the vault is to remain postoperatively where the surgeon intends it to be.

This is most easily accomplished by a transvaginal approach to surgery, as with New Orleans or McCall cul-de-plasty, but can be achieved by abdominal cul-de-plasty as well. A deep cul-de-sac should be sought out and, if found, excised or obliterated by whatever route is chosen. If the anatomic support of the vault is found to be wanting, an alternative method of support should be provided by colpopexy-sacrocolpopexy if coincident with total abdominal hysterectomy, or sacrospinous colpopexy if coincident with total vaginal hysterectomy. The surgeon should be familiar and experienced with the techniques of each operation.

An indicated hysterectomy should permit repair of any coincident cystocele, rectocele, or enterocele. The connective tissue supports to which the uterus was attached must be effectively utilized in postoperative support of the vagina, especially the vaginal vault. A pathologically wide vault should be narrowed appropriately, lessening the width of the cul-de-sac and bringing the uterosacral ligaments closer to one another and to the midline.

Some surgeons are of the view that uterine and genital prolapse are the principle indications for the vaginal approach to hysterectomy. The more experienced surgeon will recognize that, provided the uterus is movable and not larger than the size of a 12-week gestation, and that the bony pelvis of the patient is of adequate size, most hysterectomies can be done safely by the vaginal route. When prolapse is coincident, uterine descensus is the result of a genital prolapse and not the cause. The essence of surgery is to remedy the anatomic defect, here done most expeditiously by the vaginal route coincident with indicated repair work through the same operative exposure.

The degree of uterine prolapse and mobility should be estimated during the initial bimanual pelvic examination of the patient in both the lithotomy position and when standing and straining, and should be confirmed by examination under anesthesia immediately preceding hysterectomy. The presence of any genuine anatomic stress urinary incontinence should be determined so that it can be corrected simultaneous with hysterectomy by whatever route.

Possible oophorectomy should be given the same consideration whatever the route of hysterectomy, provided it can be accomplished with safety and technical precision. Generally speaking, if the ovaries are freely mobile and the infundibulopelvic ligaments are long, as follows a long-standing preoperative uterine retroversion, a transvaginal salpingo-oophorectomy can be accomplished. Even if the infundibulopelvic ligaments are short, the mesovarium, being drawn more caudally than the infundibulopelvic ligament, can be clamped under direct vision and in a majority of instances the oophorectomy done safely.

When in doubt about the exact nature of possible adnexal pathology and its contribution to inhibiting the vaginal route for surgery, a preliminary diagnostic laparoscopy will clarify the intraperitoneal state of the patient's adnexa in her pelvis. Mobility-inhibiting adhesions can be cut translaparoscopically (laparoscopic-assisted vaginal hysterectomy), and the broad ligament freed from the uterus if desired. When performed by the experienced laparoscopist, this procedure will increase the numbers of patients whose hysterectomy can be completed transvaginally, with all of the intended advantages of the latter. Rarely, the entire hysterectomy may be completed laparoscopically, but the surgeon must ensure that this approach is clearly in the best interests of the patient and does not represent a reprehensible desire of the surgeon to show off a special interest. Enthusiasm for the new must be tempered with surgical common sense. Showing that a procedure can be done using new techniques is one thing, but showing that the results are better is something else. This ethic should, of course, guide all surgical decision making and accomplishment. It is important in evaluation of laparoscopic hysterectomy to remind ourselves that the choice of such a route implies no deliberate attention to reconstructing the supports of the uterus and the vagina following hysterectomy, for which one might anticipate an increased incidence of vaginal vault prolapse in the patient predisposed to this postoperative problem.

The Transvaginal Approach

The technique of total vaginal hysterectomy is of course similar to that of total abdominal hysterectomy, but the order of the steps is reversed. When hysterectomy is done transvaginally, once the cardinal-uterosacral ligament complex has been detached from the uterus, traction to the cervix brings the uterus and its remaining attachments closer to the operator, where they too may be seen, clamped, and transsected under direct visualization. With proper technique and adequate retraction, each step of the vaginal hysterectomy can be done under the surgeon's direct vision.

The vaginal hysterectomy techniques and their many variations, once learned, are never forgotten. However, in many graduate training programs today there is insufficient instruction and practice in the field of vaginal hysterectomy and reconstructive surgery for the learner to achieve competence. This may be the result of a shortage of teachers in this area or a reluctance on the part of attending staff to attempt to develop in their juniors techniques with which they themselves are neither well versed nor comfortable. To master these techniques, whether the learner is a house officer or attending surgeon not yet experienced in this area, it is important that the gynecologist start with the easier cases, in which the technical steps are reasonably straightforward and predictable. The Heaney technique for vaginal hysterectomy is most generally chosen because of its universal safety and effective surgical result. When a number of these cases have been performed, with the best assistants available who are experienced and comfortable with the vaginal approach to surgery, the operator can begin to add the variations in technique. These will make the operation particularly well suited to those patients with additional findings that need attention (ie, obliteration or excision of the cul-de-sac of Douglas, or management of the patient with demonstratively insufficient cardinal-uterosacral ligament strength with which to support the vagina postoperatively).

Reduction in operative blood loss and operative time is directly dependent on precision in the knowledge of each patient's connective tissue septae and potential spaces. Because the blood vessels and lymphatics run in the septae, they can be identified, clamped, and cut before blood is needlessly lost. Efficiency in operating time, with the avoidance of unnecessary slowness, will not only cut down blood loss but shorten the length of operative anesthesia.

Vaginal hysterectomy is made easier by the use of instruments specifically designed for the transvaginal approach to surgery. However, it must be clearly understood that the surgeon is more important than the instruments. A good surgeon using poor instruments will obtain a better result than would a poor surgeon with good instruments. The best results, of course, come when specialized instruments are used by a skilled surgeon.

Alternatives to Hysterectomy

There are several alternates to hysterectomy currently under investigation, especially when excessive bleeding is the indication for surgery. These include transhysteroscopic endometrial ablation, either by thermocautery, laser, or resectoscope, and long-term hormone manipulation. The long-range risks and benefits will take years of observation to determine, so the field of symptom relief has never been so dynamic.

Summary

By study, practice, and constant review of results, the gynecologic surgeon not only can offer his or her patients a full spectrum of surgical options for hysterectomy, including the route for the operation itself, but also can give the patient thoughtful advice as to the reasons why a particular decision has been chosen and recommended for her surgery along with a reasonable summary of the surgeon's experience and results, the possible risks, and the planned convalescence. For most surgeons and most patients, the use of the vaginal route for hysterectomy can be increased with significant improvement in both patient comfort and cost effectiveness. This approach also will permit repair of any coincident pelvic defect. After weighing all of the options, the ideal operation will be that chosen specifically for each patient and performed correctly the first time, reducing the costly chance of future reoperation.

References

1. Copenhaver EH: Hysterectomy: Vaginal vs. abdominal. *Surg Clin North Am* 1965;45:751–753.
2. Dicker RC, Greenspan JR, Strauss LT, et al: Complications of abdominal and

vaginal hysterectomy among women of reproductive age in the United States. *Am J Obstet Gynecol* 1982;144:841–848.
3. Gitch G, Burger E, Tatra G: Trends in thirty years of vaginal hysterectomy. *Surg Gynecol Obstet* 1991;172:207–210.
4. Jeffcoate TNA (ed): *Hysterectomy and Its Aftermath: Principles of Gynaecology.* New York, Appleton-Century-Crofts, 1967, pp 929–933.
5. Nezhat C, Nezhat F, Silfen S: Laparoscopic hysterectomy and bilateral salpingo-oophorectomy using multi-fire GIA surgical stapler. *J Gynecol Surg* 1990;6:287–288.
6. Nichols DH, Randall CL: *Vaginal Hysterectomy.* ed 3. Baltimore, Williams & Wilkins Co, 1989, pp 182–237.
7. Pokras R, Hufnagel V: Hysterectomy in the United States, 1965–84. *Am J Public Health* 1988;78:852–853.
8. Ranney B: Decreasing numbers for vaginal hysterectomy and plasty. *South Dakota J Med* 1990;43:7–12.
9. Ranney B: Multiple diagnosis and procedures during hysterectomy. *Int J Gynaecol Obstet* 1990;33:325–332.
10. Reich H, DeCaprio J, McGlynn F: Laparoscopic hysterectomy. *J Gynecol Surg* 1989;5:213–216.
11. Thompson JD, Birch HW: Indications for hysterectomy. *Clin Obstet Gynecol* 1981;24:1245–1258.
12. Thompson JD: Hysterectomy, in Thompson JD, Rock JA (eds): *TeLinde's Operative Gynecology,* ed 7. Philadelphia, JB Lippincott, 1992, pp 663–738.
13. Wright RC: Hysterectomy: Past, present, and future. *Obstet Gynecol* 1969;33:560–563.

Chapter 4

Prophylactic Antibiotic Use with Elective Hysterectomy

David L. Hemsell, MD

Essentially since antibiotics were introduced into clinical medicine, surgeons have been inclined to administer antibiotics to prevent the development of infection following surgical procedures in clinically uninfected patients (prophylaxis). This practice was overutilized; many surgical procedures were associated with infection rates that were too low to justify the practice, which is not without risk. Although there is no uniform definition of an infection rate at which prophylaxis becomes indicated, reference is occasionally made to a rate of 10%. After multiple prospective, randomized, and blinded studies, it was also learned that patients did not require "prophylactic" antibiotic from the day of hospital admission through the day of discharge. More recent clinical trials have shown that a single dose of an antimicrobial agent given during the immediate preoperative period is as effective as multiple doses in preventing postoperative infection after many surgical procedures, including hysterectomy.

Hysterectomy requires transection of tissues that have a bacterial flora comprised of many significant potential pathogens for soft tissue infection and/or abscess formation. The entire surgical procedure is performed in a contaminated field during vaginal hysterectomy, whereas at abdominal hysterectomy, bacterial inoculation occurs very late in the procedure. Prospective data indicate that antimicrobial prophylaxis is indicated for women undergoing vaginal hysterectomy, but is not uniformly recommended for women undergoing abdominal hysterectomy.

Although many clinical trials conducted during the past 40 years documented the ability of antibiotics to reduce the incidence of postoperative infection, the mechanisms remain unclear. Burke[1] discovered in an animal model that maximum infection suppression resulted when there were therapeutic concentrations of antibiotic at the time of dermal incision and bacterial inoculation. If the antibiotic was not administered until 3 hours after inoculation, it was ineffective in preventing infection. This was confirmed for hysterectomy and other procedures.[2,3]

Important variables include which bacteria are present in the lower reproductive tract, their concentrations and virulence factors, duration of exposure, host resistance factors, and surgical variables such as duration of procedure, presence of blood or necrotic tissue for bacterial nutrition, and perhaps sensitivity patterns in the inoculated bacteria and the spectrum of the antibiotic administered for prophylaxis. Because of the lack of understanding of the complex pathophysiologic interaction between bacteria and the operative site/host resistance, selection of a particular antibiotic is empiric and is based on the clinical experience of the surgeon and possibly on the results of clinical trials and "guidance" from pharmaceutical representatives.

Risk Factors for Infection

Operating in a contaminated field is a universally recognized risk factor for the development of postoperative infection. Many investigators have attempted, unsuccessfully, to correlate preoperative or intraoperative cultures with the development of postoperative infection.[4-19] Postoperatively, there were increases in not only *Bacteroides* species, but also *Escherichia coli* and *Enterococcus faecalis*. Irrespective of surgical approach, these three species were frequently recovered from pelvic infection sites following hysterectomy. They were also recovered from postoperative vaginal cultures taken from many more women who did not develop infection. This fact identified a major problem that exists regarding the polymicrobial pelvic operative-site infections that develop after hysterectomy: It is impossible to identify the exact pathogens from among the flora recovered in a transvaginal culture of a pelvic infection site. Two authors recently reported that the presence of bacterial vaginosis or *Trichomonas vaginalis* in the vagina immediately prior to hysterectomy was a risk factor in the absence of prophylactic antibiotics.[20,21] They did not administer prophylaxis for those women at risk.

Unfortunately, risk factors that predict the development of operative-site infection after hysterectomy are not as universal as those predicting infections that develop after cesarean section. Many studies attempting to identify risk factors for women undergoing hysterectomy have resulted in varied results, such as patient age. In eight studies, premenopausal women were at higher risk for pelvic infection after vaginal hysterectomy,[2,22-28] but they were not at increased risk in six other clinical trials[11,29-33] or in any study addressing infection after abdominal hysterectomy. In some investigations, a longer surgery increased the risk of infection after vaginal hysterectomy[2,31-34] and abdominal hysterectomy,[2,35] but it was not associated with postoperative infection in many more clinical trials.[12,17,18,20,32,33,36-39]

When evaluated, previous surgery such as conization or dilation and curettage or additional procedures were risk factors for infection after vaginal hysterectomy in some studies,[15,26,27,31,38,40–43] but not in other studies[7,12,23,29,32,37,40,44,45] or after abdominal hysterectomy.[12,17,18,23,33] The phase of the menstrual cycle was also a risk factor for infection after vaginal hysterectomy in four clinical trials[24,29,46,47] but not in five others,[12,26,30,48,49] although it was never a risk factor when investigated with abdominal hysterectomy. In addition, excessive blood loss was a risk factor after vaginal[2,30,31,33,34,38] and abdominal[2,33] hysterectomy in some studies but not in other clinical trials in vaginal[26,29,32,38] or abdominal[17,18,20,32,36] hysterectomy.

Inexperience of the surgeon was not a risk factor for an increased incidence of infection in the majority of studies in which surgeon experience was evaluated after vaginal[7,26,33,38,50,51] or abdominal[17,18,33,52] hysterectomy. However, in one report, surgeon inexperience was a risk factor after both procedures.[25] Obesity was not a risk factor after vaginal[2,12,31,32,33,38,39] or abdominal[2,12,17,18,32,33,52] hysterectomy, except in one study of abdominal hysterectomy.[53] In contrast, lower socioeconomic status was a risk factor with vaginal[5,12,25,54,55] and abdominal[2,12,55] hysterectomy. In only one study[20] was it not identified as a risk factor.

Results of Placebo-Controlled and Comparative Antibiotic Trials

Most prospective randomized studies in which an antibiotic was compared to placebo in women undergoing vaginal hysterectomy revealed significant decreases in the infection rate with antibiotic administration. Hirsch[56] reported in a review that antibiotic prophylaxis reduced the incidence of pelvic infection from 25% to 5%. Table 4.1 lists represen-

Table 4.1 Vaginal Hysterectomy Antibiotic Prophylaxis Trials (Placebo-Controlled)

Trial	Regimen	Operative-Site Infection[a] Antibiotic	Placebo
Allen et al[50]	Cephalothin (5 days)	2/48[b] (4%)	19/50 (38%)
Ledger et al[4]	Cephaloridine (3 doses)	4/50[b] (8%)	17/50 (34%)
Breeden and Mayo[5]	Cephaloridine (3 doses)	2/54[b] (4%)	11/46 (24%)
Wright et al[57]	Neomycin/polymyxin/bacitracin vaginal spray (1 dose)	8/50[b] (16%)	17/50 (34%)
Grossman et al[12]	Cefazolin (2 days)	1/28[b] (4%)	6/24 (25%)
	Penicillin (2 days)	2/26 (8%)	
Polk et al[14]	Cefazolin (3 doses)	1/44[b] (2%)	9/42 (21%)
Hemsell et al[13]	Cefoxitin (3 doses)	4/50[b] (8%)	28/49 (57%)
Mickal et al[58]	Cefoxitin (3 doses)	7/68[b] (10%)	18/57 (32%)
Stage et al[28]	Cephradine (2 doses)	2/107[b] (2%)	8/56 (14%)

[a] Number infected/number in regimen arm; percent infected in parentheses.

[b] Significant ($p < .05$) difference in operative-site infection rates.

Table 4.2 Vaginal Hysterectomy Prospective Clinical Trials (Comparative Prophylaxis)

Trial	Regimen	Operative-Site Infection[a]
Goosenberg et al[26]	Penicillin/streptomycin (6 days)	3/40[b] (7.5%)
	Chloramphenicol (6 days)	21/40 (52.5%)
	No antibiotic	31/40 (77.5%)
Bolling and Plunkett[29]	Ampicillin (7 days) *or* Tetracycline (7 days)	5/119 (4%)
	No antibiotic	48/177[b] (27%)
Glover and van Nagell[60]	Ampicillin (7 doses)	3/100 (3%)
	Penicillin/streptomycin (3 days)	2/100 (2%)
	No antibiotic	19/100[b] (19%)
Lett et al[7]	Cefazolin (1 dose)	6/52 (12%)
	Cephaloridine (3 doses)	8/50 (16%)
	No antibiotic	31/51[b] (61%)
Peterson et al[61]	Cephalothin (3 days)	34/333[b] (10%)
	No antibiotic (Team 2)	125/398 (31%)
	No antibiotic (Team 3)	64/199 (32%)
Jacobson et al[62]	Ceforanide (2 doses)	2/76 (3%)
	Cephalothin (6 doses)	7/74 (9%)
Hemsell et al[15]	Moxalactam (3 doses)	5/93 (5%)
	Cefazolin (3 doses)	4/100 (4%)
Ferrari et al[63]	Cefazolin (3 doses)	3/62 (5%)
	Thiamphenicol (3 doses)	4/67 (6%)
	Cefazolin/thiamphenicol (3 doses)	2/66 (3%)
	No antibiotic	15/65[b] (23%)
Hemsell et al[16]	Cefoxitin (1 dose)	1/58 (2%)
	Cefoxitin (3 doses)	2/54 (4%)
Hemsell et al[64]	Ceftriaxone (1 dose)	1/64 (2%)
	Cefazolin (3 doses)	1/63 (2%)
Maki et al[65]	Cefoxitin (4 doses)	3/49 (6%)
	Cefonicid (1 dose)	0/37 (0%)
Roy and Wilkins[66]	Cefotaxime (1 dose)	1/36 (3%)
	Cefoxitin (3–5 doses)	3/38 (8%)
Benson et al[67]	Ampicillin (4 doses)	2/212 (1%)
	Ampicillin (5 days)	2/215 (1%)
Hemsell et al[31]	Ceftriaxone (1 dose)	1/57 (2%)
	Cefazolin (3 doses)	1/60 (2%)
Benigno et al[68]	Piperacillin (3 doses)	8/151 (5%)
	Cephalothin (3 doses)	5/87 (6%)
	Cefoxitin (3 doses)	3/60 (5%)
Hemsell et al[38]	Cefazolin 1 g (1 dose)	3/53 (6%)
	Cefazolin 2 g (1 dose)	2/53 (4%)
	Cefoxitin 2 g (1 dose)	2/51 (4%)
	Cefotaxime 1 g (1 dose)	3/55 (5%)
Soper and Yarwood[39]	Cefazolin (1 dose)	4/45 (9%)
	Cefazolin (3 doses)	4/45 (9%)
	Cefonicid (1 dose)	2/45 (4%)
Berkeley et al[69]	Cefotetan (1 dose)	1/70 (1%)
	Cefoxitin (3 doses)	1/33 (3%)
Hemsell et al[52]	Cefamandole (1 dose)	1/38 (3%)
	Cefotaxime (1 dose)	1/40 (2.5%)
Hager et al[70]	Mezlocillin (1 dose)	3/41 (7%)
	Cefotaxime (1 dose)	1/44 (2%)
Hemsell et al[33]	Piperacillin (1 dose)	1/52 (2%)
	Cefoxitin (3 doses)	1/51 (2%)
Roy et al[71]	Ceftizoxime (1 dose)	1/52 (2%)
	Cefoxitin (3 doses)	4/47 (9%)

(*continued*)

Table 4.2 (*continued*)

Trial	Regimen	Operative-Site Infection[a]
Multicenter Study Group[72]	Cefamandole (1 dose)	6/129 (5%)
	Cefotaxime (1 dose)	5/131 (4%)
Stiver et al[73]	Ceftriaxone (1 dose)	2/65 (3%)
	Cefazolin (3 doses)	0/73 (0%)
Hemsell et al[74]	Cefazolin (1 dose IM)	8/101 (8%)
	Cefazolin (1 dose IV)	5/106 (5%)
Mercer et al[75]	Cefonicid (1 dose)	1/50 (2%)
	Cefoxitin (4 doses)	3/50 (6%)
Regalo et al[76]	Cefotetan (1 dose)	7/246 (3%)
	Piperacillin (1 dose)	12/267 (4%)
Periti et al[77]	Cefotaxime (1 dose)	1/64 (2%)
	Cephazolin (2 doses)	5/74 (7%)
Gerger and Wilken[78]	Metronidazole (5 doses)	33/192 (17%)
	Doxycycline (2 doses)	3/116[b] (3%)
	No treatment	38/186 (20%)

[a] Number infected/number in regimen arm; percent infected in parentheses.
[b] Significant ($p < .05$) difference in operative-site infection rates.

tative prospective, randomized, placebo-controlled studies in which there was a precise definition for the type of postoperative infection. Only operative site infection data are presented. A statistically significant reduction in postoperative infection was reported, even with as few as 24 to 28 patients in comparative arms.[12]

Once it was determined that essentially all women undergoing vaginal hysterectomy benefited from prophylaxis at vaginal hysterectomy, placebo was considered to be unethical. Therefore, comparative antibiotic trials replaced placebo-controlled studies. Although a parenteral single-dose antibiotic study was reported in 1977,[7] single-dose studies were not common until the mid-1980s. It should be noted that a penicillin suppository (single-dose) was evaluated very early and found to be quite effective.[59] Table 4.2 lists representatives of studies in which pelvic infection was clearly defined. In general, one dose of antibiotic was as effective as multiple doses, and the spectrum of antibacterial activity appeared to play a small role in the protection afforded by the antibiotic. No regimen was superior to another with two exceptions.[26,78] Sample size and beta error may be important factors in these results.

Placebo-controlled antibiotic clinical trials failed to identify uniform protection against infection by the administration of prophylactic antibiotic at abdominal hysterectomy. In earlier studies, antibiotics were administered for a longer time period, as was true for vaginal hysterectomy. The lack of uniformity underscored the importance of individual determination of the need for prophylaxis in different hospital patient populations. Table 4.3 lists representative clinical trials detailing these facts. Although individual clinical trials evaluating prophylaxis at ab-

Table 4.3. Abdominal Hysterectomy Antibiotic Prophylaxis Trials (Placebo-Controlled)

		Operative-Site Infection[a]	
Trial	Regimen	Antibiotic	Placebo
Allen et al[50]	Cephalothin (5 days)	7/85[b] (8%)	18/23 (22%)
Ohm and Galask[79]	Cephaloridine/cephalexin (5 days)	4/47 (9%)	7/46 (15%)
Holman et al[80]	Cefazolin (3 doses)	3/42[b] (7%)	15/28 (39%)
Jennings[9]	Cefazolin cephalexin (7 doses +)	0/50[b] (0%)	6/52 (12%)
Grossman et al[12]	Cefazolin (2 days)	9/79 (11%)	9/84 (11%)
	Penicillin (2 days)	4/76 (5%)	
Polk et al[14]	Cefazolin (3 doses)	29/206 (14%)	47/223 (21%)
Schepars and Merkus[81]	Cefoxitin (2 doses)	3/53 (6%)	8/50 (16%)
Duff[82]	Cefoxitin (2 doses)	8/45 (18%)	12/46 (26%)
Manthorpe and Justesen[83]	Metronidazole (4 days)	14/77 (18%)	10/77 (13%)
Walker et al[84]	Metronidazole (vaginal pessary)	6/46 (13%)	6/42 (14%)
Hemsell et al[85]	Cefoxitin (3 doses)	6/50[b] (12%)	16/50 (32%)
Vincelette et al[86]	Metronidazole (3 doses)	7/53 (13%)	7/53 (13%)
Eron et al[87]	Ceftriaxone (1 dose)	2/49 (4%)	7/49 (14%)
Evaldson et al[88]	Tinidazole (1 dose)	5/49 (10%)	11/49 (22%)

[a] Number infected/number in regimen arm; percent infected in parentheses.
[b] Significant ($p < .05$) difference in operative-site infection rates.

dominal hysterectomy did not uniformly confirm benefit associated with prophylaxis, combining data from the 14 prospective studies evaluating 1,925 women (Table 4.3) provides interesting results. Even though there was a significant reduction in infection rate with antibiotic administration ranging from 1 dose to 5 days, in only 4 of the 14 (29%) trials was an overall infection rate of 10.2% observed in 1,053 women. The postoperative infection rate in the 872 women given placebo was 20.5% ($p < .001$). These combined data indicate that, indeed, prophylactic antibiotic administration will benefit women undergoing abdominal hysterectomy. The fact that there may be populations with low infection rates and no identifiable risk factors in whom the potential risks of prophylaxis would outweigh the benefits must be emphasized.

Prospective randomized comparative antibiotic clinical trials in which operative site infection was clearly defined are presented in Table 4.4. Again, no single agent proved superior with two exceptions.[96,99] Sample size may also be important here.

Additional Considerations in Prophylaxis

Financial Advantages

Davey et al[97] reported that prophylaxis given to women undergoing abdominal hysterectomy resulted in cost savings to the hospital and community health services with measurable benefits to the patient. Prophylaxis for the vaginal hysterectomy population, however, resulted in

Table 4.4 Abdominal Hysterectomy Clinical Trials (Comparative Prophylaxis)

Trial	Regimen	Operative-Site Infection[a]
Ferrari et al[63]	Cefazolin (3 doses)	8/125 (6%)
	Thiamphenicol (3 doses)	9/119 (18%)
	Cefazolin/thiamphenicol (3 doses)	4/120 (3%)
	No antibiotic	19/126[b] (15%)
Hemsell et al[17]	Cefoperazone (3 doses)	3/50 (6%)
	Cefoxitin (3 doses)	2/51 (4%)
Maki et al[65]	Cefoxitin (5 doses)	3/49 (6%)
	Cefonicid (1 dose)	0/37 (0%)
Poulsen et al[89]	Metronidazole (oral, 2 doses)	1/50[b] (2%)
	Suction drainage	6/50 (12%)
	Control	9/50 (18%)
Roy and Wilkins[66]	Cefotaxime (1 dose)	5/55 (9%)
	Cefoxitin (3–5 doses)	6/35 (17%)
Berkeley et al[90]	Moxalactam (3 doses)	4/50 (8%)
	Cefazolin (3 doses)	3/50 (6%)
	No antibiotic	2/50 (4%)
Hemsell et al[18]	Cefoxitin (1 dose)	2/50 (4%)
	Cefoxitin (2 doses)	6/50 (12%)
	Cefoxitin (3 doses)	2/50 (4%)
Hemsell et al[31]	Ceftriaxone (1 dose)	4/54 (7%)
	Cefazolin (3 doses)	4/59 (7%)
Tuomala et al[91]	Cefazolin (3 doses)	6/108 (6%)
	Moxalactam (3 doses)	6/100 (6%)
Senior and Steigrad[92]	Cefoxitin (3 doses)	1/61 (2%)
	Cephradine/tinidazole (1 dose)	0/59 (0%)
	No antibiotic	5/65[b] (8%)
Berkeley et al[69]	Cefotetan (1 dose)	9/157 (6%)
	Cefoxitin (3 doses)	4/78 (5%)
Hemsell et al[52]	Cefamandole (1 dose)	6/79 (8%)
	Cefotaxime (1 dose)	2/84 (2%)
Hemsell et al[33]	Piperacillin (1 dose)	3/51 (6%)
	Cefoxitin (3 doses)	2/53 (4%)
Hemsell et al[74]	Cefazolin (1 dose IM)	20/264 (8%)
	Cefazolin (1 dose IV)	21/275 (8%)
Berkeley et al[93]	Cefotetan (1 dose)	7/88 (8%)
	Cefoxitin (3 doses)	4/40 (10%)
Mercer et al[75]	Cefotetan (1 dose)	2/92 (2%)
	Piperacillin (1 dose)	6/81 (7%)
Periti et al[94]	Cefotetan (1 dose)	4/11 (3%)
	Cefazolin (2 doses)	2/124 (2%)
McDonald et al[95]	Cefotaxime (1 dose)	4/96 (4%)
	Cefotaxime (8 doses)	4/84 (5%)
Periti et al[77]	Cefotaxime (1 dose)	9/138 (7%)
	Cefazolin (2 doses)	13/139 (9%)
Brown et al[96]	Amoxicillin/clavulanic acid (3 doses)	3/130[b] (2%)
	Metronidazole (3 doses)[c]	16/138 (12%)
Davey et al[97]	Cephradine (1 dose)	16/97 (16%)
	Mezlocillin (1 dose)	23/101 (23%)
	Placebo (1 dose)	29/102 (29%)

(continued)

Table 4.4 (continued)

Trial	Regimen	Operative-Site Infection[a]
Eron et al[98]	Cefonicid (1 dose)[d]	4/91 (4%)
	Cefonicid (1 dose)[e]	2/33 (6%)
	Cefoxitin (5 doses)	2/33 (6%)
Mele et al[99]	Cefazolin (15 doses)	8/70 (11%)
	Cefamandole (6 doses)	15/120 (12.5%)
	Ceftriaxone (1 dose)	6/180[b] (3%)

[a] Number infected/number in regimen arm; percent infected in parentheses.
[b] Significant ($p < .05$) difference in operative-site infection rates.
[c] Suppository.
[d] Given 3.5–5 hours preoperatively.
[e] Given 0.5–1 hour preoperatively.

increased cost to the hospital, no savings to community services, and no significant benefit to the patient. Cost considerations are receiving increased emphasis. An operative site infection increases hospital costs by at least $1,500, and in many instances by considerably more. This fact is a strong argument for prophylaxis, especially when added to patient morbidity that may be prevented by prophylaxis.

Hospitals that have infection control or morbidity surveillance teams are well equipped to make individual determinations about the necessity for prophylaxis, the true incidence of symptomatic or asymptomatic temperature elevation, the incidence of postoperative infection (both operative site and distant), the efficacy of various regimens for prophylaxis, and the efficacy of regimens given for therapy of postoperative infections. Unbiased surveillance is very important! It is hoped that, in the future, all hospitals will have the luxury of such surveillance teams.

Incidence of Distant Infection

The incidence of atelectasis, pneumonia, and phlebitis are essentially unaltered by prophylaxis at hysterectomy.[12] There are data indicating that prophylactic administration of antibiotic at hysterectomy will significantly reduce not only operative site infection, but also urinary tract infection in those patient populations having a high incidence of that postoperative infection. The incidence of such infections in patients in our hospital is so low that antibiotic prophylaxis has never had an impact on them. In one study, McDonald et al[95] reported that 4 days of antibiotic administration was superior to single-dose or short-course prophylaxis in the prevention of urinary tract infection.

Route of Administration

It was established in our patient population that route of administration had no impact on prophylactic efficacy.[74] For that reason, and to prevent the potential scenario in which a patient received an intramuscular dose on the ward and did not have surgery, we elect to administer prophylactic antibiotic intravenously in the operating room after the intravenous line is placed. If the infusion is initiated prior to anesthesia, the patient can identify an adverse reaction early before the dose is completely administered, thereby potentially resulting in a less severe reaction. Between 10% and 15% of the patients in our prospective antibiotic studies admit allergy to penicillin; the manifestation is usually rash or hives. We have administered parenteral cephalosporin to those patients without allergic manifestation. We have on occasion observed allergic reactions in non–penicillin-allergic women given multiple-dose cephalosporin after the first dose, however.

Advantages of Single-Dose Prophylaxis

Administration of any antibiotic is associated with some risk. The most potentially life-threatening of these risks is anaphylaxis. Obviously, the more doses administered, the greater the theoretic likelihood for that or any other adverse result, such as induction of bacterial resistance. We have observed that as few as three prophylactic doses of antibiotic do significantly alter not only the bacteria that are recovered from the lower reproductive tract postoperatively, but also their resistance patterns. Such changes are not observed after a single dose. Colonic bacteria are also more likely to be altered by multiple doses of antibiotic, which may result in either antibiotic-associated diarrhea or pseudomembranous enterocolitis. Other obvious advantages of single-dose prophylaxis include decreased cost, decreased nursing service time, and a decrease in other ancillary costs such as intravenous tubing and minisacs.

Recommendations

Because of the current cost of cefazolin, and a lack of definitive proof that there is a more effective agent for prophylaxis, cefazolin is most commonly recommended for prophylaxis. A large prospective, randomized, and blinded prophylaxis study evaluating over 1,000 women undergoing hysterectomy is currently underway to ascertain whether an agent with an expanded spectrum of both aerobic and anaerobic antibacterial activity offers enhanced protection over that provided by cefazolin. Although the second-generation cephalosporin may cost six times more per gram than cefazolin, the prevention of a single infection would pay for the antibiotic cost difference for between 100 and 200 women undergoing hysterectomy. Cefazolin remains a logical choice for hysterectomy prophylaxis until a superior regimen is identified. No data show that a 2-g dose is superior to a 1-g dose. Unless individual evaluation identifies a subset of women who benefit from a second dose, a single preoperative 1-g dose of cefazolin provides cost-effective, efficient infection protection.

References

1. Burke JF: The effective period of preventive antibiotic action in experimental incisions and dermal lesions. *Surgery* 1961;50:161–168.
2. Shapiro M, Munoz A, Tager IB, et al: Risk factors for infection at the operative site after abdominal or vaginal hysterectomy. *N Engl J Med* 1982;307:1661–1666.
3. Classen DC, Evans RS, Pestotnik SL, et al: The timing of prophylactic administration of antibiotics and the risk of surgical-wound infection. *N Engl J Med* 1992;326:281–286.
4. Ledger WJ, Sweet RL, Headington JT: Prophylactic cephaloridine in the treatment of postoperative pelvic infection in premenopausal women undergoing vaginal hysterectomy. *Am J Obstet Gynecol* 1973;115:766–774.
5. Breeden JT, Mayo JE: Low dose prophylactic antibiotics in vaginal hysterectomy. *Obstet Gynecol* 1974;43:379–385.
6. George JW, Ansbacher R, Otterson WN, et al: Prospective bacteriologic study of women undergoing hysterectomy. *Obstet Gynecol* 1975;45:60–63.
7. Lett WJ, Ansbacher R, Davison BL, et al: Prophylactic antibiotics for women undergoing vaginal hysterectomy. *J Reprod Med* 1977;19:51–54.
8. Grossman JH III, Adams RL, Hierholzer WJ Jr, et al: Endometrial and vaginal cuff bacteria recovered at elective hysterectomy during a trial of antibiotic prophylaxis. *Am J Obstet Gynecol* 1978;130:312–316.
9. Jennings RH: Prophylactic antibiotics in vaginal and abdominal hysterectomy. *South Med J* 1978;71:251–254.
10. Grossman JH III, Adams RL: Vaginal flora in women undergoing hysterectomy with antibiotic prophylaxis. *Obstet Gynecol* 1979;53:23–26.
11. Mendelson J, Portnoy J, De Saint Victor JR, et al: Effect of single and multidose cephradine prophylaxis on infectious morbidity of vaginal hysterectomy. *Obstet Gynecol* 1979;53:31–35.
12. Grossman JH III, Greco TP, Minkin MJ, et al: Prophylactic antibiotics in gynecologic surgery. *Obstet Gynecol* 1979;53:537–544.
13. Hemsell DL, Cunningham FG, Kappus S, et al: Cefoxitin for prophylaxis in premenopausal women undergoing vaginal hysterectomy. *Obstet Gynecol* 1980;56:629–634.
14. Polk BF, Shapiro M, Goldstein P, et al: Randomized clinical trial of perioperative cefazolin in preventing infection after hysterectomy. *Lancet* 1980;1:437–441.
15. Hemsell D, Hemsell P, Nobles B, et al: Moxalactam versus cefazolin prophylaxis for vaginal hysterectomy. *Am J Obstet Gynecol* 1983;147:379–385.
16. Hemsell DL, Heard ML, Nobles BJ, et al: Single-dose cefoxitin prophylaxis for premenopausal women undergoing vaginal hysterectomy. *Obstet Gynecol* 1984;63:285–290.
17. Hemsell DL, Johnson ER, Bawdon RE, et al: Cefoperazone and cefoxitin prophylaxis for abdominal hysterectomy. *Obstet Gynecol* 1984;63:467–472.
18. Hemsell DL, Hemsell PG, Heard ML, et al: Preoperative cefoxitin prophylaxis for elective abdominal hysterectomy. *Am J Obstet Gynecol* 1985;153:225–226.
19. Smith CV, Gallup DG, Gibbs RL, et al: Oral doxycycline vs. parenteral cefazolin: Prophylaxis for vaginal hysterectomy. *Infect Surg* 1989;99:64–67.

20. Soper DE, Bump RC, Hurt WG: Bacterial vaginosis and trichomoniasis vaginitis are risk factors for cuff cellulitis after abdominal hysterectomy. *Am J Obstet Gynecol* 1990;163:1016–1023.
21. Larsson P-G, Platz-Christensen J-J, Forsum U, et al: Clue cells in predicting infections after abdominal hysterectomy. *Obstet Gynecol* 1991;77:450–452.
22. Taylor ES, Hansen RR: Morbidity following vaginal hysterectomy and colpoplasty. *Obstet Gynecol* 1961;17:346–348.
23. Maudsley RF, Robertson EM: Common complications of hysterectomy. *Can Med Assoc J* 1965;92:908–911.
24. Pratt JH, Galloway JR: Vaginal hysterectomy in patients less than 36 or more than 60 years of age. *Am J Obstet Gynecol* 1965;93:812–821.
25. Hall WL, Sobel AI, Jones CP, et al: Anaerobic postoperative pelvic infections. *Obstet Gynecol* 1967;30:1–7.
26. Goosenberg J, Emich JP Jr, Schwarz RH: Prophylactic antibiotics in vaginal hysterectomy. *Am J Obstet Gynecol* 1969;105:503–506.
27. Boyd ME, Garceau R: The value of prophylactic antibiotics after vaginal hysterectomy. *Am J Obstet Gynecol* 1976;125:581–585.
28. Stage AH, Glover DD, Vaughan JE: Low-dose cephradine prophylaxis in obstetric and gynecologic surgery. *J Reprod Med* 1982;27:113–119.
29. Bolling DR Jr, Plunkett GD: Prophylactic antibiotics for vaginal hysterectomies. *Obstet Gynecol* 1973;41:689–692.
30. Sprague AD, van Nagell JR Jr: The relationship of age and endometrial histology to blood loss and morbidity following vaginal hysterectomy. *Am J Obstet Gynecol* 1974;118:805–808.
31. Hemsell DL, Johnson ER, Bawdon RE, et al: Ceftriaxone and cefazolin prophylaxis for hysterectomy. *Surg Gynecol Obstet* 1985;161:197–203.
32. Wijma J, Kauer FM, van Saene HKF, et al: Antibiotics and suction drainage as prophylaxis in vaginal and abdominal hysterectomy. *Obstet Gynecol* 1987;70:384–388.
33. Hemsell DL, Johnson ER, Heard MC, et al: Single-dose piperacillin versus triple-dose cefoxitin prophylaxis at vaginal and abdominal hysterectomy. *South Med J* 1989;82:438–442.
34. Fleming SP, Kerns PR, Locke FR: Factors influencing morbidity following vaginal hysterectomy. *Obstet Gynecol* 1954;4:295–301.
35. Ledger WJ, Campbell C, Willson JR: Postoperative adnexal infections. *Obstet Gynecol* 1968;31:83–89.
36. Roy S, Wilkins J: Comparison of cefotaxime and cefazolin for prophylaxis of vaginal or abdominal hysterectomy. *Clin Ther* 1982;5(suppl A):74–82.
37. Hemsell DL, Hemsell PG, Nobles BJ: Doxycycline and cefamandole prophylaxis for premenopausal women undergoing vaginal hysterectomy. *Surg Gynecol Obstet* 1985;161:462–464.
38. Hemsell DL, Bawdon RE, Hemsell PG, et al: Single-dose cephalosporin for prevention of major pelvic infection after vaginal hysterectomy: Cefazolin versus cefoxitin versus cefotaxime. *Am J Obstet Gynecol* 1987;156:1201–1205.
39. Soper DE, Yarwood RL: Single-dose antibiotic prophylaxis in women undergoing vaginal hysterectomy. *Obstet Gynecol* 1987;69:879–882.
40. Cavanagh D, Rutledge F: The cervical cone biopsy-hysterectomy sequence and factors affecting the febrile morbidity. *Am J Obstet Gynecol* 1960;80:53–59.

41. Malinak LR, Jeffrey RA Jr, Dunn WJ: The conization-hysterectomy time interval: A clinical and pathologic-study. *Obstet Gynecol* 1964;23:317–329.
42. DeCenzo JA, Malo T, Cavanagh D: Factors affecting cone-hysterectomy morbidity: A study of 200 patients. *Am J Obstet Gynecol* 1971;110:380–384.
43. van Nagell JR Jr, Roddick JW Jr, Cooper RM, et al: Vaginal hysterectomy following conization in the treatment of carcinoma in-situ of the cervix. *Am J Obstet Gynecol* 1972;113:948–951.
44. Cron RS, Stauffer J, Paegel H Jr: Morbidity studies in 1000 consecutive hysterectomies. *Am J Obstet Gynecol* 1952;63:344–350.
45. Coulam CB, Pratt JH: Vaginal hysterectomy: Is previous pelvic operation a contraindication? *Am J Obstet Gynecol* 1973;116:252–260.
46. Neary MP, Allen J, Okubadejo OA, et al: Preoperative vaginal bacteria and postoperative infections in gynaecological patients. *Lancet* 1973;2:1291–1294.
47. Thadepalli H, Savage EW Jr, Salem FA, et al: Cyclic changes in cervical microflora and their effect on infections following hysterectomy. *Gynecol Obstet Invest* 1982;14:176–183.
48. Tashjian JH, Coulam CB, Washington JA II: Vaginal flora in asymptomatic women. *Mayo Clin Proc* 1976;51:557–561.
49. Levison ME, Corman LC, Carrington ER, et al: Quantitative microflora of the vagina. *Am J Obstet Gynecol* 1977;127:80–85.
50. Allen JL, Rampone JF, Wheeless CR: Use of a prophylactic antibiotic in elective major gynecologic operations. *Obstet Gynecol* 1972;39:218–224.
51. Kuhn RJP: Chemoprophylaxis with tinidazole in major gynaecological surgery. *Aust N Z J Obstet Gynaecol* 1980;20:43–46.
52. Hemsell DL, Hemsell PG, Nobles BG, et al: Single-dose cefamandole and cefotaxime prophylaxis at vaginal and abdominal hysterectomy. *Adv Ther* 1988;5:97–102.
53. Pitkin RM: Abdominal hysterectomy in obese women. *Surg Gynecol Obstet* 1976;142:532–536.
54. White SC, Wartel LJ, Wade ME: Comparison of abdominal and vaginal hysterectomies: A review of 600 operations. *Obstet Gynecol* 1971;37:530–537.
55. Ledger WJ, Child MA: The hospital care of patients undergoing hysterectomy: An analysis of 12,026 patients from the Professional Activity Study. *Am J Obstet Gynecol* 1973;117:423–433.
56. Hirsch H: Prophylactic antibiotics in obstetrics and gynecology. *Am J Med* 1985;78:170–176.
57. Wright VC, Lanning NM, Natale R: Use of a topical antibiotic spray in vaginal surgery. *Can Med Assoc J* 1978;118:1395–1398.
58. Mickal A, Curole D, Lewis C: Cefoxitin sodium: Double-blind vaginal hysterectomy prophylaxis in premenopausal patients. *Obstet Gynecol* 1980;56:222–225.
59. Turner SJ: The effect of penicillin vaginal suppositories on morbidity in vaginal hysterectomy and on the vaginal flora. *Am J Obstet Gynecol* 1950;60:806–812.
60. Glover MW, van Nagell JR Jr: The effect of prophylactic ampicillin on pelvic infection following vaginal hysterectomy. *Am J Obstet Gynecol* 1976;126:385–388.
61. Peterson LF, Justema EJ, Wiersma AF, et al: Comparative efficacy of pre-

operative and postoperative cephalothin therapy in vaginal hysterectomy. *Curr Ther Res* 1977;22:792–797.
62. Jacobson JA, Hebertson R, Kasworm E: Comparison of ceforanide and cephalothin prophylaxis for vaginal hysterectomies. *Animicrob Agents Chemother* 1982;22:643–647.
63. Ferrari A, Baccolo M, Privitera G, et al: Randomized clinical trial of short-term antibiotic prophylaxis in 750 patients undergoing vaginal and abdominal hysterectomy. *Int Surg* 1984;69:21–27.
64. Hemsell DL, Menon MO, Friedman AJ: Ceftriaxone or cefazolin prophylaxis for the prevention of infection after vaginal hysterectomy. *Am J Surg* 1984; 148:22–26.
65. Maki DG, Lammers JL, Aughey DR: Comparative studies of multiple dose cefoxitin vs. single-dose cefonicid for surgical prophylaxis in patients undergoing biliary tract operations or hysterectomy. *Rev Infect Dis* 1984; 6(suppl 4):S887–S895.
66. Roy S, Wilkins J: Single-dose cefotaxime versus 3 to 5 dose cefoxitin for prophylaxis of vaginal or abdominal hysterectomy. *J Antimicrob Chemother* 1984;14(suppl B):217–221.
67. Benson WL, Brown RL, Schmidt PM: Comparison of short and long courses of ampicillin for vaginal hysterectomy. *J Reprod Med* 1985;30:874–878.
68. Benigno BB, Evrard J, Faro S, et al: A comparison of piperacillin, cephalothin and cefoxitin in the prevention of postoperative infections in patients undergoing vaginal hysterectomy. *Surg Gynecol Obstet* 1986;163:421–427.
69. Berkeley AS, Freedman KS, Ledger WJ, et al: Comparison of cefotetan and cefoxitin prophylaxis for abdominal and vaginal hysterectomy. *Am J Obstet Gynecol* 1988;158:706–709.
70. Hager WD, Sweet RL, Charles D, et al: Comparative study of mezlocillin versus cefotaxime single-dose prophylaxis in patients undergoing vaginal hysterectomy. *Curr Ther Res* 1989;45:63–69.
71. Roy S, Wilkins J, Hemsell DL, et al: Efficacy and safety of single-dose ceftizoxime vs. multiple-dose cefoxitin in preventing infection after vaginal hysterectomy. *J Reprod Med* 1988;33(suppl):149–153.
72. Multicenter Study Group: Single-dose prophylaxis in patients undergoing vaginal hysterectomy: Cefamandole versus cefotaxime. *Am J Obstet Gynecol* 1989;160:1198–1201.
73. Stiver HG, Binns BO, Brunham RC, et al: Randomized, double-blind comparison of efficacies, costs, and vaginal flora alterations with single-dose ceftriaxone and multidose cefazolin prophylaxis in vaginal hysterectomy. *Antimicrob Agents Chemother* 1990;34:1194–1197.
74. Hemsell DL, Johnson ER, Hemsell PG, et al: Cefazolin for hysterectomy prophylaxis. *Obstet Gynecol* 1990;76:603–606.
75. Mercer LJ, Murphy HJ, Ismail MA, et al: A comparison of cefonicid and cefoxitin for preventing infections after vaginal hysterectomy. *J Reprod Med* 1988;33:223–226.
76. Regallo M, Scalambrino S, Negri L, et al: Cefotetan versus piperacillin in the prophylaxis of abdominal and vaginal hysterectomy: A prospective randomized study. *Drugs Exp Clin Res* 1989;XV(6/7):315–320.
77. Periti P, Mazzei T, Orlandini F, et al: Comparison of the antimicrobial prophylactic efficacy of cefotaxime and cephazolin in obstetric and gynaeco-

logical surgery. A randomised multicentre study. *Drugs* 1988;35(suppl 2): 133–138.
78. Gerger VB, Wilken H: Effektivitat der perioperativen Antibiotikaprophylaxe mit Metronidazol oder Doxycyclin bei der vaginalen Hysterektomie. *Zentralbl Gynakol* 1989;111:1542–1548.
79. Ohm MJ, Galask RP: The effect of antibiotic prophylaxis on patients undergoing total abdominal hysterectomy. I. Effect on morbidity. *Am J Obstet Gynecol* 1976;125:442–454.
80. Holman JF, McGowan JE, Thompson JD: Perioperative antibiotics in major elective gynecologic surgery. *South Med J* 1978;71:417–420.
81. Schepars JP, Merkus FHM: Cefoxitin sodium: Double-blind, placebo-controlled, prophylactic study in premenopausal patients undergoing abdominal hysterectomy. *Clin Pharmacol Ther* 1981;29:281–286.
82. Duff P: Antibiotic prophylaxis for abdominal hysterectomy. *Obstet Gynecol* 1982;60:25–29.
83. Manthorpe T, Justesen T: Metronidazole prophylaxis in abdominal hysterectomy: A double-blind controlled study. *Acta Obstet Gynecol Scand* 1982;61:243–246.
84. Walker EM, Gordon AJ, Warren RE, et al: Prophylactic single-dose metronidazole before abdominal hysterectomy. *Br J Obstet Gynaecol* 1982;89:957–961.
85. Hemsell DL, Reisch J, Nobles B, et al: Prevention of major infection after elective abdominal hysterectomy: Individual determination required. *Am J Obstet Gynecol* 1983;147:520–528.
86. Vincelette J, Finkelstein F, Aoki FY, et al: Double-blind trial of perioperative intravenous metronidazole prophylaxis for abdominal and vaginal hysterectomy. *Surgery* 1983;93:185–189.
87. Eron LJ, Saltzman D, Sites J: Prophylaxis of infection following abdominal hysterectomy by ceftriaxone: A placebo-controlled trial, in *25th Interscience Conference of Antimicrobial Agents and Chemotherapy, Program and Abstracts,* P301, #1141. Washington, DC, American Society of Microbiology, 1985.
88. Evaldson GR, Lindgren S, Malmborg AS, et al: Single-dose intravenous tinidazole prophylaxis in abdominal hysterectomy. *Acta Obstet Gynecol Scand* 1986;65:361–365.
89. Poulsen HK, Borel J, Olsen H: Prophylactic metronidazole or suction drainage in abdominal hysterectomy. *Obstet Gynecol* 1984;63:291–294.
90. Berkeley AS, Hayworth SD, Hirsch JC, et al: Controlled comparative study of moxalactam and cefazolin for prophylaxis of abdominal hysterectomy. *Surg Gynecol Obstet* 1985;161:457–461.
91. Tuomala RE, Fischer SG, Munoz A, et al: A comparative trial of cefazolin and moxalactam as prophylaxis for preventing infection after abdominal hysterectomy. *Obstet Gynecol* 1985;66:372–376.
92. Senior CC, Steigrad SJ: Are preoperative antibiotics helpful in abdominal hysterectomy? *Am J Obstet Gynecol* 1986;154:1004–1008.
93. Berkeley AS, Orr JW, Cavanagh D, et al: Comparative effectiveness and safety of cefotetan and cefoxitin as prophylactic agents in patients undergoing abdominal or vaginal hysterectomy. *Am J Surg* 1988;155(5A):81–85.
94. Periti P, Mazzei T, Periti E: Prophylaxis in gynaecological and obstetric sur-

gery: A comparative randomised multicentre study of single-dose cefotetan versus two doses of cefazolin. *Chemioterapia (International Journal of the Mediterranean Society of Chemotherapy)* 1988;7:245–252.
95. McDonald PJ, Sanders R, Turnidge J, et al: Optimal duration of cefotaxime prophylaxis in abdominal and vaginal hysterectomy. *Drugs* 1988;35(suppl 2):216–220.
96. Brown EM, Depares J, Robertson AA, et al: Amoxycillin-clavulanic acid (Augmentin) versus metronidazole as prophylaxis in hysterectomy: A prospective, randomized clinical trial. *Br J Obstet Gynaecol* 1988;95:286–293.
97. Davey PG, Duncan ID, Edward D, et al: Cost-benefit analysis of cephradine and mezlocillin prophylaxis for abdominal and vaginal hysterectomy. *Br J Obstet Gynaecol* 1988;95:1170–1177.
98. Eron LJ, Gordon SF, Harvey LK, et al: A trial using early preoperative administration of cefonicid for antimicrobial prophylaxis with hysterectomies. *DICP* 1989;23:655–658.
99. Mele G, Loizzi P, Greco P, et al: Antibiotic prophylaxis for abdominal hysterectomy. *Clin Exp Obstet Gynecol* 1988;4:154–156.

Chapter 5

Urinary and Intestinal Tract Injuries

Donald G. Gallup, MD

Most injuries to the lower urinary tract occur during the course of gynecologic-related procedures, usually hysterectomy. Of all genitourinary fistulas in the Mayo Clinic series, 74% of the patients had benign conditions. Of the vesicovaginal fistulas in this series, the causative procedure was a "simple" abdominal hysterectomy in 70% of the patients.[1] Similarly, ureterovaginal injuries occur in a large percentage of patients who have hysterectomy for benign disease, although they may have preexisting conditions such as endometriosis or tuboovarian abscesses, which distort the normal anatomy. Bowel injuries associated with surgery are also frequently associated with similar preexisting conditions of endometriosis, pelvic inflammatory disease, inflammatory bowel disease, prior irradiation, or a history of multiple previous abdominal operations.

The primary goal of this chapter is to familiarize the gynecologist with preventative methods to avoid each of these injuries. If an injury occurs, recognition of it using immediate and delayed techniques will be emphasized. Finally, the management of injuries and their sequelae will be presented.

Bladder Injuries

An unrecognized bladder injury will result in fistula formation. In the United States, reports in the last two decades indicate that over 80% of bladder injuries are associated with gynecologic surgery. Less frequent causes (around 5% each) include irradiation, obstetric trauma, various urologic procedures, and trauma.[1–3] Of note, in third world countries, particularly in Africa, obstetrically related incidents continue to be the major cause of vesicovaginal fistulas (VVFs). Most of these obstetric fistulas are due to prolonged obstructed labor causing pressure necrosis. One contributing factor, particularly in northern Nigeria, is marriage at a very young age (10 to 12 years), with subsequent childbirth before the pelvis is completely formed. Female circumcision plays an etiologic role in some cultures. *Yankan gishiri,* practiced by Hausa women in Nigeria, is still done. The procedure, done by "witches" and sometimes midwives, consists of a vertical cut to the pubic bone in the anterior vaginal wall and is done for a variety of reasons.[4-6] Attitudes toward women with these fistulas is harsh, and the vast majority of such women are eventually abandoned.

Vesicovaginal fistulas associated with hysterectomy are predominately abdominal procedures. For instance, in the recent Mayo Clinic data of 156 women with VVFs, 85% had had abdominal hysterectomies, 13% had had vaginal hysterectomies, and only 2% had had a radical hysterectomy.[1]

Prevention of Injuries

Most bladder injuries resulting in subsequent fistula formation can be prevented. Surgeons should ensure that a Foley catheter has been inserted prior to performing "crash" cesarean sections. During hysterectomy, the bladder should be initially separated from the cervix by sharp dissection, whether the hysterectomy is vaginal or abdominal. During vaginal hysterectomy, we prefer to incise and ligate the bladder pillars in order to avoid bladder injury and injury to the uterus. Large-bore sutures and large clamps should be avoided when in close proximity to the bladder or ureters. Cautery, particularly near the base of the bladder, should also be avoided.

Repair of Injuries

Whenever a bladder injury is suspected, the bladder should be distended with a dilute colored dye such as indigo carmine or methylene blue. (Sterile milk may also be used and has the advantage of being nonstaining.) One way to accomplish this is by simply attaching a 50-mL syringe with adaptor to the Foley and pouring the solution (300 to 400 mL) into the separated syringe. If the injury is posterior, the space of Retzius should be developed (Figure 5.1). A vertical incision can then be made in the dome of the bladder, and the trigone can be visualized. If the laceration is within 1 cm of the trigone, a no. 6 to 8 French feeding tube or ureteral catheter should be placed prior to repair in order to avoid injury.

We prefer to close an injury or large cystotomy in two layers. Preferably, the edges of the bladder should be grasped initially with Allis clamps. A through-and-through (serosa to mucosa, mucosa to serosa) running suture of 2-0 chromic is used. A second layer of interrupted 2-0 polyglycolic acid sutures is added (Figure 5.2). Some surgeons prefer to avoid including the mucosa in first layer, which is the reason we use readily absorbable chromic. Failure to include the mucosa may result in troublesome postoperative hematuria. If the laceration is near the tri-

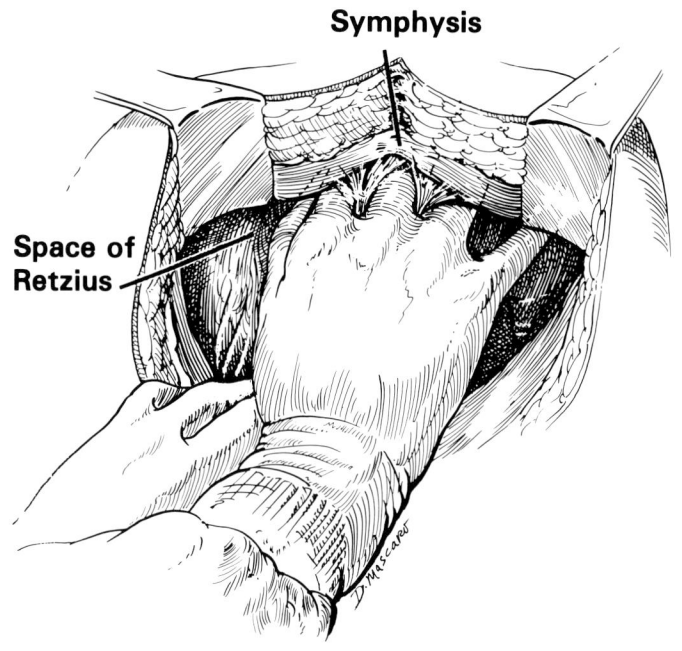

Figure 5.1 Development of the space of Retzius. The weight of the surgeon's hand in the *midline* separates the bladder from the overlying symphysis. The bladder can then be mobilized. *Reprinted, by permission, from Gallup DG, Talledo OE: Diagnosis and management of the patient with a fistula, in Phelan JP, Clark SL (eds): Cesarean Delivery. New York, Elsevier Science Publishing Co, Inc, 1988, pp 449–461.*

gone, we prefer to use a suprapubic catheter. The retroperitoneal space is drained with a closed drainage system (Jackson-Pratt or Blake) until the bladder catheter is removed, in 3 to 7 days, depending on the size of the injury.

Fistulas

Symptoms and Diagnosis

An "unrecognized" injury usually presents as a VVF with a variety of accompanying symptoms, ranging from episodic dampness with position change to constant watery discharge. Patients with a vesicouterine fistula may have cyclic hematuria. Those with a vesicoenteral fistula may have fecaluria or pneumaturia.

Two office procedures can aid in the diagnosis of urinary tract fistulas. To detect the site of a fistula, insert sterile milk into the bladder and inject 5 mL of indigo carmine dye intravenously. If the fluid in the vagina is white on speculum visualization, the patient probably has a VVF. If it is blue, she probably has ureterovaginal fistula. If it is powder-blue or white and blue, she may have both. One can also use the three-tampon technique of Moir to detect very small fistulas.[7] The patient is placed in

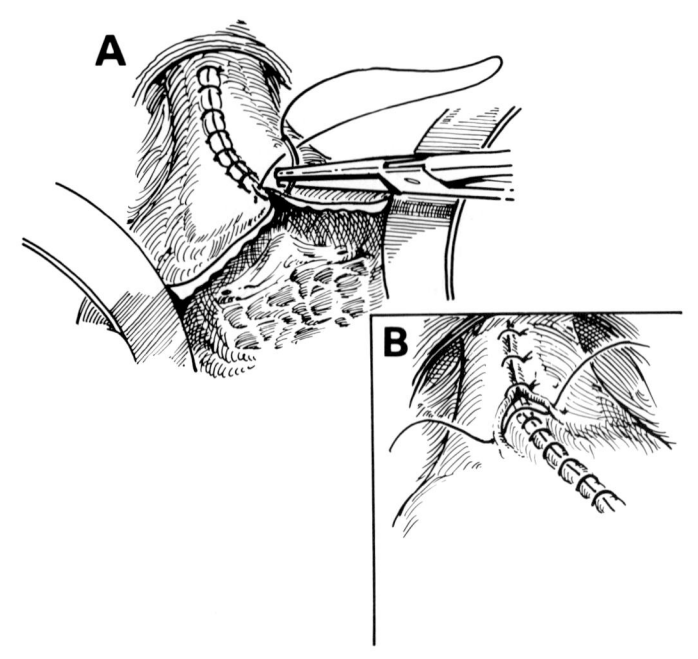

Figure 5.2 Closure of bladder injuries. **A.** A running suture of 2-0 chromic is used for the first layer of closure. **B.** The second layer is closed with interrupted 2-0 polyglycolic acid. *Reprinted, by permission, from Gallup DG, Talledo OE: Diagnosis and management of the patient with a fistula, in Phelan JP, Clark SL (eds): Cesarean Delivery. New York, Elsevier Science Publishing Co, Inc, 1988, pp 449–461.*

the dorsal lithotomy position, and three large dry cotton balls (tampons) are inserted into the vagina. The bladder is distended with dilute methylene blue dye. If the upper tampon is wet only and not blue, the patient probably has a ureterovaginal fistula. If the middle tampon is blue, she probably has a VVF. If the most distal one is blue, she may have a urethrovaginal fistula. Sometimes patients may be asked to ambulate with the tampons inside in order to detect minuscule fistulas. Evaluation of the upper tract is always indicated, even with a small VVF, and an intravenous pyelogram (IVP) and possibly a retrograde pyelogram are needed.

Occasionally, other tests may be indicated in small or more unusual fistulas. Cystoscopy in the knee-chest position or insertion of a small amount of air into the vagina with a cystoscope in place may allow one to see small bubbles rise in the fluid-filled bladder. A cystogram with a lateral view may be of aid, and a delayed voiding cystogram may detect a small vesicouterine fistula, if contrast is seen in the uterus. Vesicouterine fistulas can also be confirmed with a hysterosalpingogram. Diagnostic tests to detect vesicoenteral fistulas include ingestion of Congo red dye or charcoal, cystogram, barium enema, or upper gastrointestinal series with small bowel follow-through.

Timing of Repair

The timing of repair of a simple VVF should be determined on an individual basis. It depends on the cause, size, and site of the fistula. An empiric 6-month wait for all patients with VVF is inappropriate. Collins and associates[8,9] have advocated oral cortisone to improved local inflammation and allow early repair. Most of their patients were successfully operated within 30 days of diagnosis, and one third were operated within 14 days. Certainly, large or complicated fistulas should not be repaired early, and most experienced fistula surgeons prefer to delay intervention until local tissue reactions have ceased, usually at 4 to 6 months. Most obstetrically related fistulas may also require a 4- to 6-month delay to allow involution of tissues in the birth canal.

Recent reports indicate that small, uncomplicated fistulas associated with surgery (usually hysterectomies) can be safely closed 8 weeks after injury.[10-13] Teasing the tissue with an Allis clamp may help determine when edema and inflammation have resolved. We prefer to wait at least 6 weeks, even with surgically related fistulas. Spontaneous closure following catheterization with an indwelling Foley has been noted in 10% to 20% of VVF patients.[14-16] Most fistulas that close spontaneously are millimeter size and usually close within 3 weeks. A conservative trial of catheter drainage is indicated at least for that period of time.

Surgical Considerations

According to Moir,[7] over 95% of VVFs can be repaired using a vaginal approach. Whether these are closed transabdominally or transvaginally, a ureteral catheter should be placed prior to surgical intervention if the ureteral orifices are within 1 cm of the fistulous tract or if the fistula is sufficiently large that the integrity of the ureter might be compromised during repair. In postmenopausal women, or women who are estrogen deficient for other reasons, topical estrogen should be applied at least 3 weeks prior to repair. All patients are placed on prophylactic antibiotics. Because tissues may be more vascular and engorged during menstruation, making dissection more difficult, the time chosen for surgical intervention should be well away from the menstrual period. Although cortisone, given 7 to 10 days preoperatively, may help decrease edema more quickly,[8,9] the possibility of impaired wound healing makes its use controversial.

Latzko Partial Colpocleisis

Most gynecologists use the transvaginal approach. The vast majority of VVFs in the United States are associated with prior hysterectomies and are usually small to medium sized. Many gynecologists use the Latzko technique of partial colpocleisis to repair these uncomplicated fistulas.[14,17,18]

Positioning of patients is critical for adequate exposure. For the

Latzko procedure, the exaggerated lithotomy position with moderate Trendelenburg tilt gives adequate exposure in most patients. The exaggerated lithotomy position implies that the patient's buttocks protrude over the end of the table. About 15° of Trendelenburg tilt will allow the anterior vaginal wall to appear perpendicular to the surgeon's line of vision. In patients with small-caliber vaginas, a Schucardt's incision should be employed. Large labia should be stitched laterally. Neosynephrine (1:200,000) injected into the fistula site will facilitate dissection and decrease blood loss. Vasopressin (Pitressin), 10 units (1 ampule) in 50 mL of saline, is an alternate solution.

A small-caliber Foley catheter is inserted into the fistula to help provide traction. Additionally, four-quadrant traction sutures of 0 silk or polypropylene are placed to aid in traction, allowing the surgeon to pull the fistula to the operating field. A circular area around the tract is removed in four quadrants, using a no. 11 blade (Figure 5.3). The fistulous tract is not removed. The area over the fistula is closed in an inverting manner, using interrupted 3-0 polyglycolic acid suture.

We prefer the use of a suprapubic catheter. The length of urinary drainage depends on the size of the fistula and the quality of tissues encountered during repair. The tissues heal slowly, and rarely is the

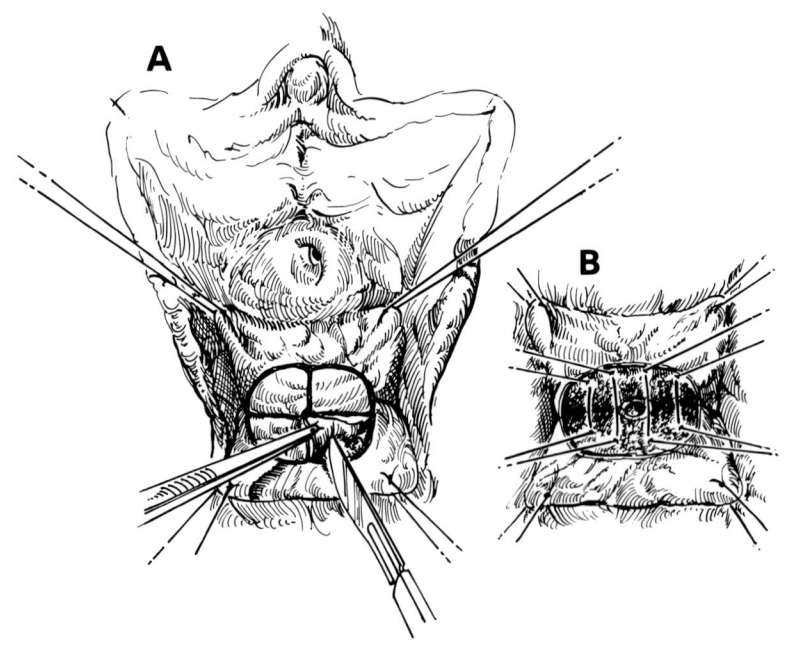

Figure 5.3 Latzko partial colpocleisis technique. **A.** The vaginal mucosa surrounding the fistula is removed in quadrants. **B.** The vagina is approximated over the intact tract with layers of 3-0 polyglycolic acid interrupted sutures. *Reprinted, by permission, from Gallup DG, Talledo OE: Diagnosis and management of the patient with a fistula, in Phelan JP, Clark SL (eds): Cesarean Delivery. New York, Elsevier Science Publishing Co, Inc, 1988, pp 449–461.*

period of drainage less than 10 days. Some leave the catheter only until the urine is grossly cleared of blood (as little as 2 to 3 days). However, a failed repair must be avoided, and a few extra days of catheterization can be tolerated by most patients. The patient is instructed to avoid coitus for 8 weeks.

Other Repair Techniques

For *large fistulas,* better exposure may be achieved by placing the patient in the prone position with the ankles raised by stirrups (the Lawson position).[19] After obtaining appropriate exposure and injecting vasopressin solution, the junctional zone between the bladder and vagina is incised. The key to successful repair is adequate mobilization of tissues by use of a no. 11 blade or Mayo scissors (Figure 5.4). Special attention must be given to the lateral extensions of the fistula. All palpable adhesive bands are carefully divided, regardless of the size of the fistula. Thus, flaps of vaginal tissue are created. Most surgeons only freshen the fistula tract, and scar excision is unnecessary (Figure 5.5). The bladder is closed without tension. All sutures of 3-0 polyglycolic acid for each layer must be placed and tied from lateral to medial or anterior to posterior, depending on the ease of approximation of the tissue in individual patients. Two to three layers should be used.[19-23] Most of these large fistulas will

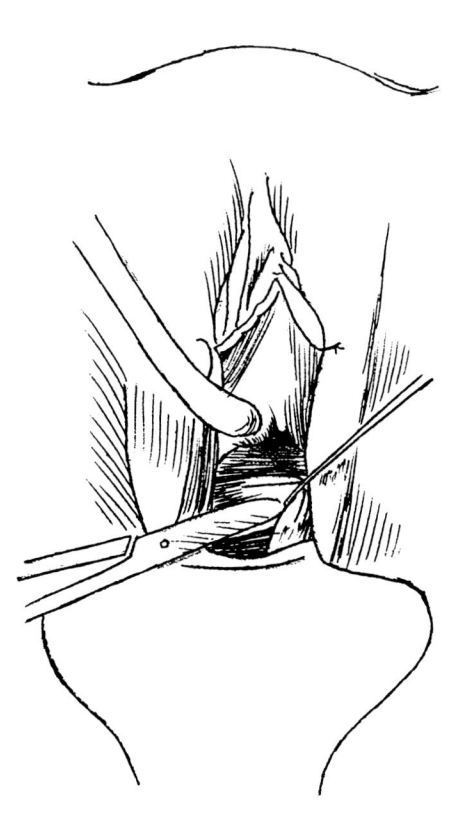

Figure 5.4 Mobilization of tissues for repair of large fistula. Countertraction is applied with a skin hook. The bladder and vagina are widely separated from each other with the use of scissors.

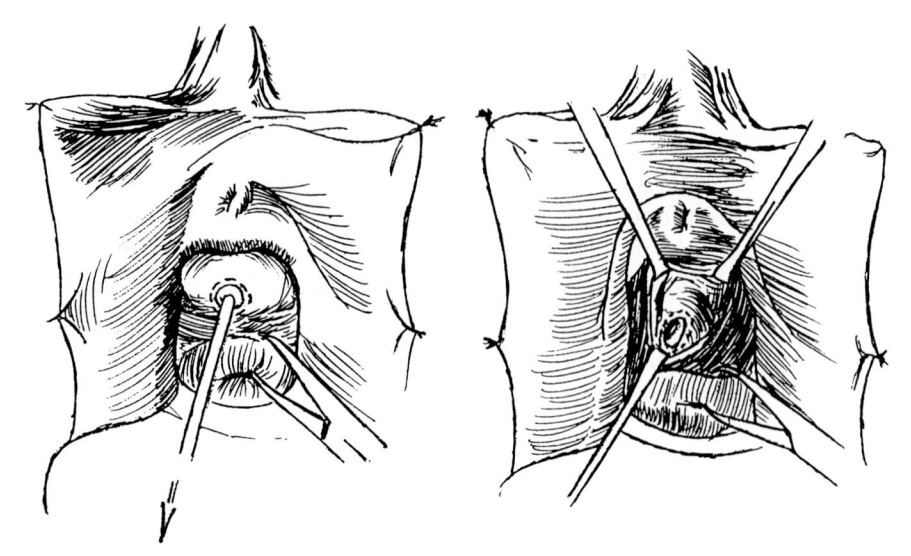

Figure 5.5 Left: A vesicovaginal fistula associated with pregnancy is pulled into the operating field with a pediatric Foley. **Right:** Wide mobilization has been done and flaps created. The area within the dotted line is not excised; the bladder is closed in layers over the intact tract. The created vaginal flaps can be tailored for close approximation without redundant tissue.

require ureteral catheterization to avoid injury. A suprapubic catheter should be left in place for a minimum of 2 weeks. We prefer to use a loosely placed vaginal pack for 48 hours, particularly when some type of graft is used as described below. If ureteral catheters are used, they should be left for 7 to 10 days.

Suprapubic extraperitoneal, transvesical, and transabdominal procedures have a limited place in repairing obstetrically related or vault fistulas. There are few contraindications to transvaginal repair. Most of them are relative (Table 5.1).

To augment transvaginal repairs of large VVFs or fistulas involving

Table 5.1 Contraindications to Transvaginal Closure of Vesicovaginal Fistula

Absolute Contraindications
Complex fistulas involving bowel or uterus
Ureteral involvement
Inaccessible location of fistula
Contracted bladder that requires patching

Relative Contraindications
Large fistula
Multiple prior repairs
Fistulas associated with radiation therapy
Excessive vaginal scarring

the urethra, *local grafts of tissue* from the labia, gracilis muscle, or portions of the gluteus maximus have been used. The use of the bulbocavernosus graft has been credited to Martius and was introduced to the United States in the English translation of Martius' *Operative Gynecology*.[24] Boronow[25] has used the Martius technique to successfully close 50% of radiation-induced VVFs. According to Betson,[26] the graft has four functions: (1) adds support to the urethral neck, (2) adds bulk to the bladder neck and bladder base, (3) decreases and/or obliterates the dead space between vaginal mucosa and bladder, and (4) brings in a new blood supply to an area of poor vascularity. The labial fat pad is available in most patients. Because its blood supply is from the external and internal pudendal arteries, the labial fat pad graft can be mobilized from anterior or posterior.[27] With radiation-induced VVFs, we prefer to use a modified bulbocavernosus myocutaneous flap, as suggested by Hoskins et al.[28] In their technique, a small skin island was kept intact with the underlying fibrofatty tissue.

According to O'Conor,[29] the key to *successful abdominal closure* of difficult VVFs is bisection of the bladder to the fistula, with wide mobilization of the bladder and vagina in separate planes. The dome of the bladder is opened, and a vertical incision is carried down to the fistula. The tract is excised and the vagina is closed separately. Fat, peritoneum, abdominal musculature, or omentum is placed between the bladder and vagina. The bladder is closed separately. A suprapubic catheter is preferred.

Ureteral Injuries

Ureteral injuries are usually associated with pelvic surgical procedures. Their incidence varies from 0.4% to 2.5% of all gynecologic procedures.[1,30-32] Because only about one third of ureteral injuries are recognized, this estimated incidence is probably low. In the Mayo Clinic series, surgical procedures for benign conditions were responsible for 27 of 31 ureterovaginal fistulas. Abdominal hysterectomy was associated with 15 of these and vaginal hysterectomy with nine.[1] Unrecognized ureteral injury can result in eventual loss of the kidney in as many as 25% of cases.

Prevention

Recognizing the patient at risk for injury will help prevent injuries and their later complications. Patients at risk might have one or several of the conditions noted in Table 5.2. Of note, gynecologists, not gynecologic oncologists, will be operating on the vast majority of patients, as indicated in the table. Preoperative evaluation with IVPs is indicated in patients with these preexisting conditions. With regard to preoperative ureteral catheterization in such patients, we are opposed for the following

Table 5.2 Conditions Associated with Ureteral Injury

1. Large adherent pelvic mass
2. Intraligamentary leiomyomata
3. Induration of paracervical tissue
    a. Infection
    b. Cancer[a]
4. Ureteral anomalies
5. Extensive pelvic inflammatory disease
6. Endometriosis
7. Prior pelvic surgery
8. Prior pelvic radiation therapy[a]

[a] Patients with these preexisting conditions usually will be operated on by gynecologic oncologists.

reasons: (1) intraoperative manipulation against the catheter can damage the mucosa of the ureter; (2) in cases of fibrosis resulting from infection, irradiation, or endometriosis, the ureter still sometimes cannot be palpated; and (3) if doubt exists about the ureter's location, it can always be cannulated during the procedure. Ureteral duplication may be an indication, if the orifices can be visualized during cystoscopy.

The ureter is only 1.5 cm lateral to the cervix and is most commonly injured where it passes under the uterine artery. Other sites of injury include the infundibulopelvic ligament at the pelvic brim and distally, close to the ureteroversical junction. One can avoid intraoperative injury in high-risk patients by entering the peritoneum laterally prior to ligating the infundibulopelvic ligament. This maneuver can be done by palpating the external iliac artery and psoas muscle and opening the peritoneum directly over the vessel. The ureter can then be palpated and visualized on the medial leaf of the broad ligament. In cases of intraligamentary fibroids, the ureter must be separated from the leiomyoma and visualized to its insertion into the tunnel. Wide bladder mobilization is indicated in selected patients to avoid distal injuries. Large clamps and massive ligatures should be avoided in this area. Indiscriminate use of cautery also should be avoided. As pointed out by many, the ureter can also be palpated during vaginal procedures.[33] This maneuver is of particular value in the patient with uterine prolapse.

Intraoperative Diagnosis and Repair

If suspicion of a ureteral injury during an operation is raised, intraoperative evaluation is mandatory. The step-by-step evaluation process might include:

1. Injection of methylene blue or indigo carmine dye directly into the ureter with concomitant proximal pressure. One carefully observes the course of the ureter for extravasation. This technique is valuable

in detecting "crush" injuries or transection, but not for inadvertent ligation.

2. With no appearance of dye in the peritoneal cavity, a cystotomy should be done after mobilizing the space of Retzius (Figure 5.1). The vertical incision is started in the dome of the bladder, and the trigone is exposed. An alternate procedure for orifice visualization is the use of suprapubic teloscopy, as recently reported by Timmons and Addison.[34]

3. Indigo carmine dye (5 mL) is injected intravenously (IV), and the ureteral orifices are observed for the efflux of blue dye, usually occurring 3 to 5 minutes later. Urinary output can be increased by injecting 12.5 mg of mannitol IV prior to injecting the dye.

4. If no efflux is noted, a no. 6 to 8 French ureteral catheter (or pediatric feeding tube) is passed retrogradely with the aid of a grooved Campbell's ureteral catheter passer (Figure 5.6).

5. If the catheter cannot be passed from below, a stab wound is made and the catheter is passed caudad into the bladder. The stab wound site should be where the ureter is usually easily located, at the bifurcation of the common iliac vessels.

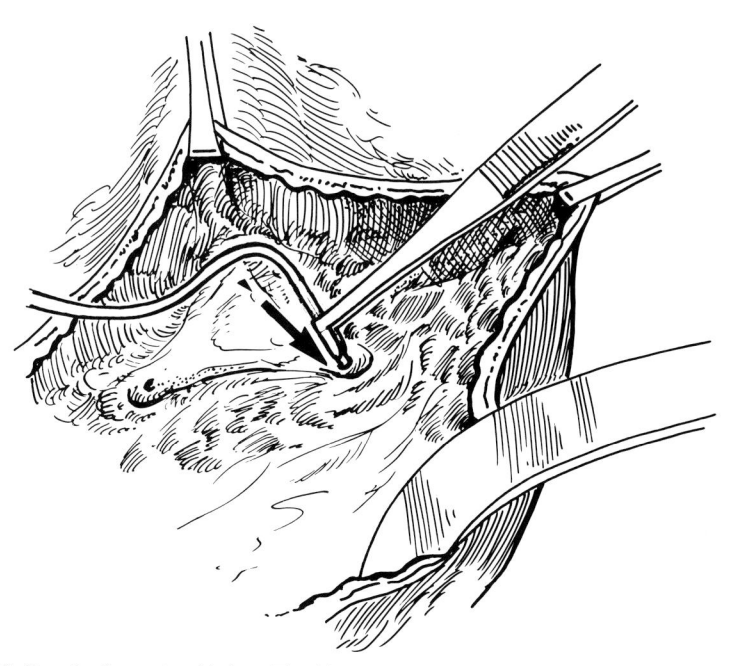

Figure 5.6 Repair of a ureteral injury. The bladder has been opened and the trigone visualized. A Campbell's ureteral catheter passer is used to pass a no. 6 to 8 French catheter retrogradely (*arrow*) through the left ureteral orifice. *Reprinted, by permission, from Gallup DG, Talledo OE: Diagnosis and management of the patient with a fistula, in Phelan JP, Clark SL (eds): Cesarean Delivery. New York, Elsevier Science Publishing Co, Inc, 1988, pp 449–461.*

In the event of suspected injury during vaginal procedures, cystoscopy should be done, indigo carmine dye injected IV, and the orifices observed. A noninvasive method to detect ureteral injuries is the use of an *intraoperative* IVP.

The "crush" or ligature injury should be managed by injecting indigo carmine dye IV. If there is extravasation at the suspected injury site, the areas should be resected and repaired. With no extravasation, a no. 6 to 8 French ureteral catheter or pediatric feeding tube can be used as a splint. A soft retroperitoneal drain should be placed close to the injury site. Partial transections can be managed with interrupted through-and-through sutures (serosa-muscularis-mucosa to mucosa-muscularis-serosa) of 4-0 chromic or polyglycolic acid. The lacerated areas should be splinted and a retroperitoneal drain utilized. Repair of major recognized injuries is basically the same as repair for "unrecognized" injuries and will be outlined below.

"Unrecognized" Ureteral Injury

Diagnosis

Most of the diagnostic techniques noted in the discussion of bladder injuries apply to ureteral injuries as well. The IVP is the mainstay of postoperative diagnosis. In one patient who had "ascites" postoperatively, we made the diagnosis of ureteral injury by paracentesis and the use of IV indigo carmine dye. Cystoscopy and retrograde pyelography are often needed to determine the exact location of the lesion or obstruction. Classic symptoms of fever, chills, flank pain, and passage of urine through the vagina, skin, or rectum should lead to the initiation of these diagnostic tests. Some patients with prior ureteral injuries may present with abdominal distention, "ascites," paralytic ileus, incontinence, or even a mass—the pseudocystic urinoma.

Timing of Repair

The timing of repair of "unrecognized" injuries is controversial. Most of the techniques for ureteral reconstruction require a lengthy operation, and the patient's general condition has an important bearing on when repairs should be attempted. Immediate repair (1 to 30 days) has been utilized with few complications.[35–37] Tarkington et al[38] believes that injuries associated with gynecologic surgery can be safely managed without delayed surgery. They noted no serious postoperative sequelae in patients with ureteral reconstruction done on an average of 6 days after initial surgery. However, in general, repair of injuries diagnosed after 72 hours is postponed for 4 to 6 weeks because of edema and associated local inflammation.

If a Silastic catheter can be passed at the time of retrograde studies, obstruction can be circumvented in some patients. Often a percutaneous nephrostomy can be done and the small catheter passed beyond the obstruction or laceration.[39–43] As many as 15% of ureteral fistulas will heal spontaneously if a ureteral catheter can be left in place for 7 to 10 days.[42–44] Our practice is to intervene in a period less than 6 weeks after injury only if retrograde catheterization or stenting is unsuccessful and if percutaneous nephrostomy cannot be done. Periodic (every 4 weeks) renal sonograms should be done to evaluate the upper tract, because worsening of obstructive uropathy may be an indication for earlier surgical intervention.

Surgical Considerations

If the fistula has not healed within a period of several months, or if there is progressive deterioration of renal function, operative repair is indicated. The surgeon must adhere to the time-honored principles of repair, whether the injury is repaired immediately or delayed repair is utilized. These include maintenance of hemostasis, use of a limited number of sutures to avoid necrosis, ureteral catheterization and retroperitoneal drainage, and absolute lack of tension at the anastomotic site. The type of repair depends on the site and the extent of injury[45] (Table 5.3).

Ureteroneocystostomy

We prefer the open technique of reanastomosing the ureter to the bladder for distal injuries. The distal ureter is ligated with permanent sutures and the bladder is mobilized from its anterior attachments (Figure 5.1). A vertical incision is made in the dome of the bladder. A small incision is made on the side of injury, and a fine-tipped clamp is pushed through the serosa. The ureter is brought into the bladder and spatulated (Figure 5.7). The spatulated ends are sutured to the bladder mucosa and muscularis with 4-0 chromic or polyglycolic acid suture. If a single-J ureteral catheter is unavailable, we prefer to place a 4-0 chromic suture through the ureter and a no. 6 to 8 French pediatric feeding tube at the level of the pelvic brim to ensure the splint is not displaced by ureteral peristalsis. Three or four sutures of 3-0 nylon or polypropylene are placed through the outside bladder wall and the ureteral adventitia at the anastomotic

Table 5.3 General Types of Ureteral Repair

1. Below midpelvis (within 4–6 cm of ureterovesicle junction)—ureteroneocystotomy
2. Above midpelvis—ureteroureterostomy
3. Above midpelvis—extensive injury
   a. Transureteroureterostomy
   b. Mobilization of kidney and ureter
   c. Ureteroileocystoplasty
   d. Cutaneous ureterostomy

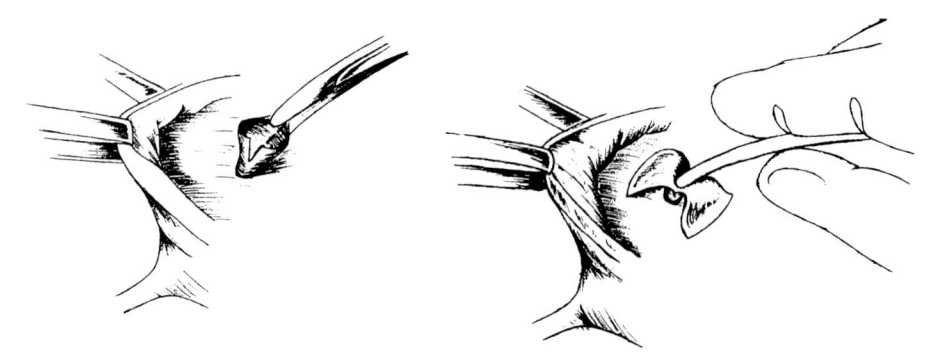

Figure 5.7 Ureteroneocystotomy. **Left:** The ureter has been pulled into the bladder and is spatulated. **Right:** A no. 6 to 8 French pediatric feeding tube is passed cephalad to the renal pelvis.

site to ensure stability and a tension-free anastomosis. The ureteral catheter is brought out through a separate stab wound in the bladder and abdomen and tied to a suprapubic catheter. The ureteral and suprapubic catheters are removed in 10 to 14 days in nonirradiated patients.

The use of a submucosal tunnel is controversial, and many surgeons advocate direct, open implantation in the dome area.[46–48] Wheeless,[49] noting that the adult urinary tract system is unique, found more long-term complications in patients who had tunneling procedures, compared to those who had direct implantation. Tunneling is time consuming in an emergency situation because it requires a relatively long ureter, and its use may result in scarring.

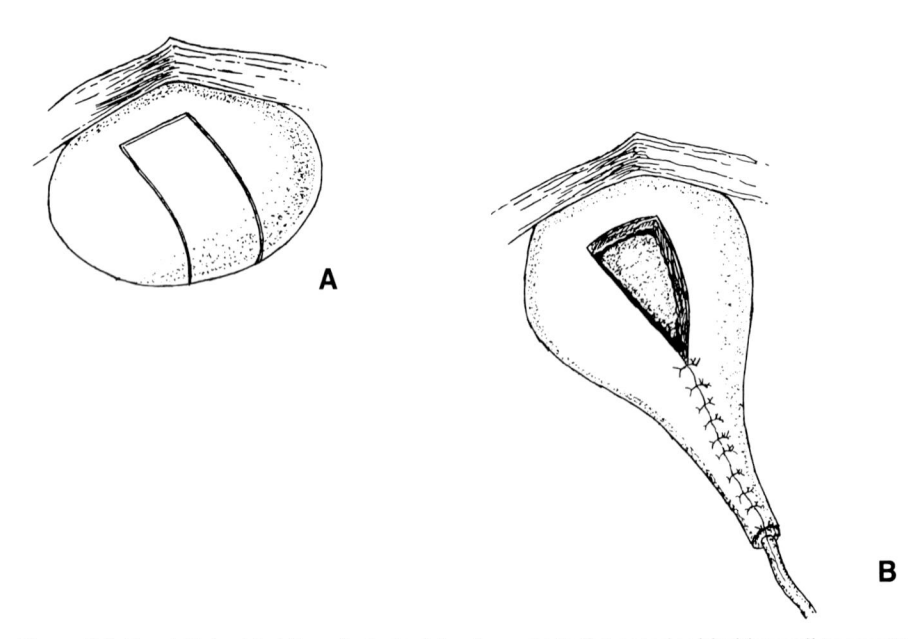

Figure 5.8 Boari-Ockerblad flap. **A.** An incision is made in the anterior bladder wall to create a flap. **B.** A tube is thus created that can be reanastamosed to the ureter.

DEMEL

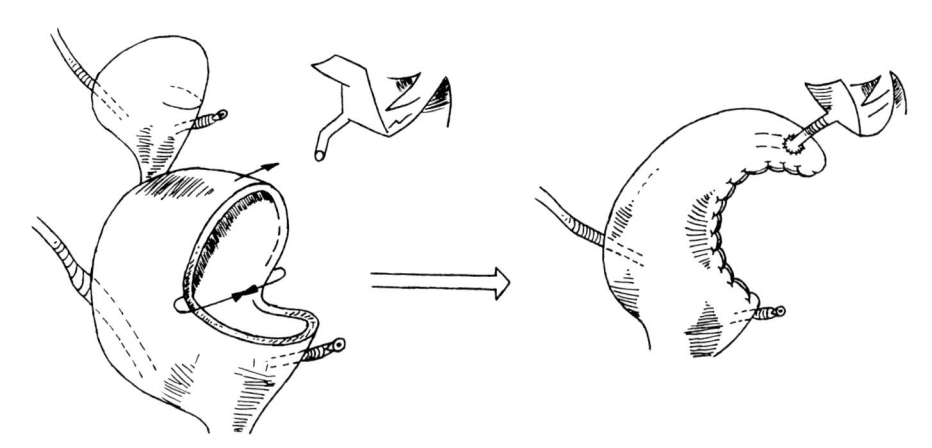

Figure 5.9 Demel technique. The bladder is sectioned transversely and sutured longitudinally. The ureter is reunited to the "new dome."

When the ureteral injury is below the pelvic brim and the ureter appears to be too short for a tension-free reanastomosis, a psoas muscle hitch for the mobilized bladder can be used.[50] Three or four permanent sutures are used to attach the seromuscular layers of the bladder to the ipsilateral psoas muscle belly. When a long segment of distal ureter is involved, the gap can be bridged by utilizing a flap from the bladder, as described in the Boari-Ockerblad method[51] (Figure 5.8). The Demel technique[52] (bladder splitting) is an excellent alternative because it is less prone to stricture development, and is our flap of choice (Figure 5.9).

Ureteroureterostomies

For minimally involved injuries above the pelvic brim, an end-to-end ureteroureterostomy can be done. The damaged area must be excised. The ureter should be mobilized from the pelvic peritoneum to ensure the proposed anastomosis is tension free. The ureter should be spatulated, one segment anteriorly and one posteriorly, or a Z-plasty done to create a larger lumen. We prefer to insert a no. 6 to 8 French urethral catheter before repair. Four through-and-through sutures are used; all layers are incorporated with 4-0 polyglycolic acid (Figure 5.10). A vertical ureterostomy, about 2 cm in length and 5 cm cephalad to the anastomosis, is advocated.[30,43,53] Some believe the anastomotic site should be reinforced with omental fat.[30,54] A soft, retroperitoneal closed drainage system, placed away from the suture area, is left in place as long as the ureteral catheter (14 to 21 days), or until the drainage is less than 30 mL in 24 hours.

Mobilization of the ipsilateral kidney may be necessary to reduce

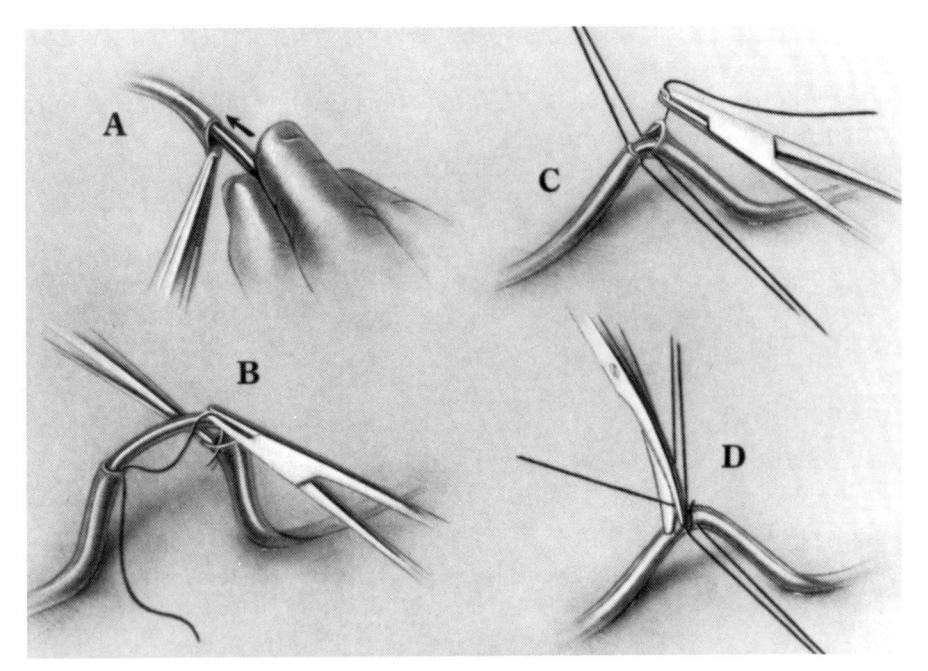

Figure 5.10 Ureteroureterostomy. A catheter is inserted into the ureter. A through-and-through suture (knot on outside) of 4-0 polyglycolic acid is first placed posteriorly. Only four sutures are used. *Reprinted, by permission, from Talledo OE, Gallup DG: Manual on Surgical Techniques. Augusta, The Medical College of Georgia, 1988, p 45.*

tension. Transureteroureterostomy is a valuable option when a large segment of ureter has been injured.[30] The proximal ureter is tunneled retroperitoneally across the midline and sutured to the contralateral ureter. This procedure can be associated with stenosis, leakage, and possible damage to the intact urinary system. Another option is inserting the ureter into a segment of small intestine, which is then sutured to the bladder (ureteroileocystoplasty). A urologist or gynecologic oncologist should be consulted for these procedures. With large defects above the pelvic brim and lack of expertise, or if the patient is unstable, any gynecologist is capable of performing a cutaneous ureterostomy.[45] A no. 6 to 8 French catheter (fixed with a suture) is inserted into the ureter and brought out retroperitoneally through a stab wound in the abdominal wall. A closed drainage system should be placed at the injury site. This is preferable, by far, to ligation of the ureter and its later consequences.

Bowel Injuries

Intestinal tract injuries during gynecologic surgery are potentially lethal. The vast majority of lacerations of the bowel during gynecologic surgery occur when the peritoneum is entered or while one is lysing bowel adhesions. However, they also occur during vaginal surgery and at the time of dilatation and curettage. We have noticed an apparent increase in bowel injuries during laparoscopy. Occasionally, a late-occurring bowel complication can be the result of an inappropriately placed suture during closure of the abdomen.

Bowel complications can be divided into those that require emergency repair (e.g., lacerations or obstruction) and those that require later intervention after work-up (eg, fistulas or intractable rectal bleeding). They can also be divided into small and large bowel injuries and their sequelae. The latter are divided into those occurring above or below the peritoneal reflection.

Prevention

As with patients with urinary tract injuries, certain patients are at risk for small and large bowel injuries (Table 5.4). As also noted for the urinary tract, the only condition the general gynecologist is not likely to encounter is prior radiation therapy. Patients with these preexisting conditions should be given some type of bowel preparation when elective surgery is contemplated. We prefer the 1-day whole gut lavage with Golytely solution (Table 5.5). Some surgeons prefer not to use antibiotics.

Tips for avoiding bowel injury during abdominal surgery are listed in Table 5.6. One must be particularly careful in using any blunt dissection

Table 5.4 Conditions Associated with Bowel Injuries

1. Endometriosis
2. Prior surgery or abdominal trauma
3. Pelvic inflammatory disease
4. History of appendicitis
5. Granulomatous pelvic disease
6. Inflammatory bowel disease
7. Prior abdominal/pelvic radiation therapy[a]

[a] These patients usually will be operated on by gynecologic oncologists.

Table 5.5 Modified 1-Day Whole Gut Lavage with Golytely Solution

1. Two days prior to operation, give patient 1 oral bisacodyl tablet to be taken at home hs.
2. One day prior to operation:
   a. Clear liquid diet
   b. Begin chilled Golytely PO at 0900 h. The rate of ingestion should be 1.2–1.8 L/h for a total of 3–8 h.
   c. Golytely is discontinued when clear liquid passes per rectum.
   d. Neomycin sulfate, 1 g PO at 1300, 1400, and 2300 h.
   e. Erythromycin base, 1 g PO at 1300, 1400, and 2300 h.
   f. No enemas are needed.
3. Day of surgery:
   a. Fleet's enema at 0630 h.
   b. Cefoxitin sodium may be given: 2 g IV push on call and 2 g IV push q6h × 3.

For patients who cannot tolerate Golytely, the solution may be infused via a nasogastric tube.

Table 5.6 Avoiding Bowel Injury during Abdominal Surgery

1. Open the abdomen cephalad to prior incisions.
2. Enter the peritoneum with a knife
3. Use traction, countertraction, and sharp dissection when separating bowel loops.
4. Dissect bowel loops one at a time.
5. "Stay out of the hole." Dissect deeper bowel loops during the last steps in lysing adhesions.
6. Avoid the use of lap pads or sponges to handle previously irradiated bowel.

on bowel mesentery. A nasogastric tube should be placed during any bowel surgery in order to avoid distention. To avoid bowel injuries during laparoscopy, patients with suspected adhesive disease may be candidates for open laparoscopy. If a perforation is suspected during dilatation and curettage, one should not proceed with curetting.

Repairing Superficial and Minor Injuries

In general, nonirradiated bowel serosal tears do not need repair. To assess bowel viability in suspected mesentery vascular injuries or multiple serosal tears, the affected areas may simply be covered with wet, warm lap pads and the bowel reassessed for appropriate color and peristalsis after a period of 10 to 15 minutes.

For small puncture injuries, a pursestring suture is often adequate. This can be done with 3-0 silk, polypropylene, or nylon (Figure 5.11).

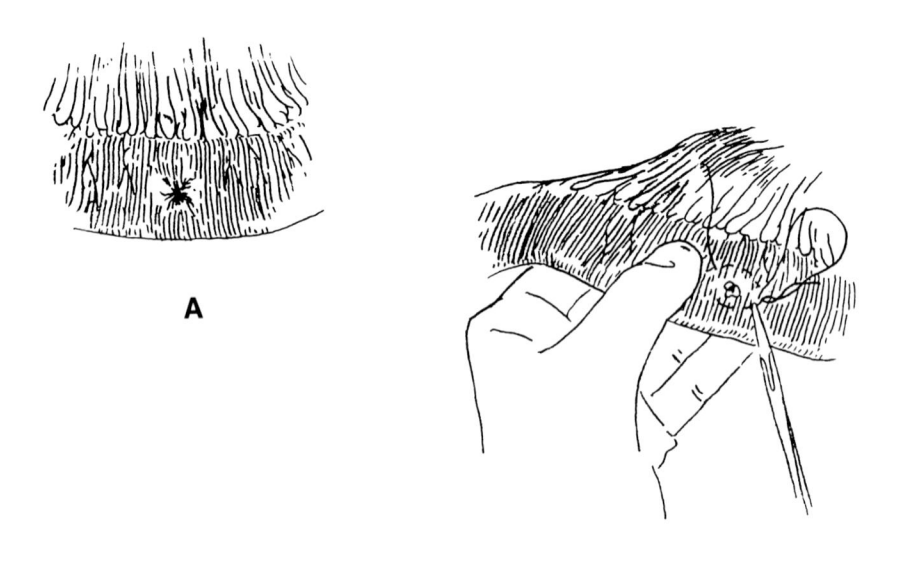

Figure 5.11 A small puncture injury of the bowel **(A)** is sutured with a pursestring technique after stabilization of the bowel with the surgeon's hand **(B)**.

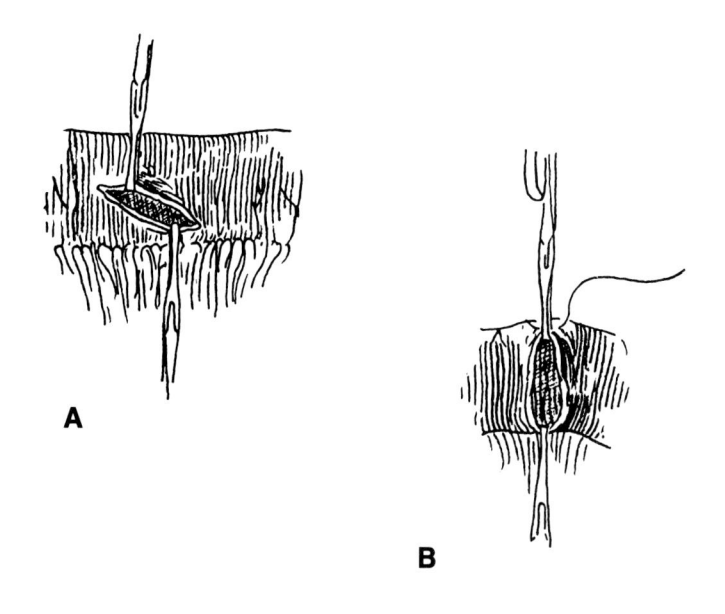

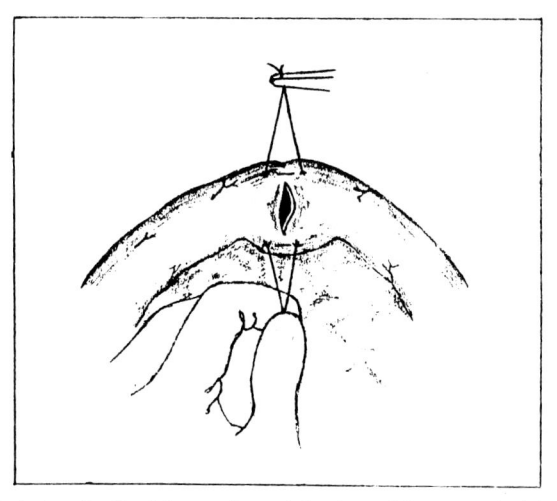

Figure 5.12 A longitudinal laceration of the bowel is converted to a horizontal laceration prior to repair. This can be done with traction sutures.

Some gynecologic surgeons are "timid" about obtaining adequate serosal bites. The serosal bites should include the muscularis. It is preferable to enter the lumen of the bowel with a needle than to use a superficial bite that simply tears through the serosa on tying.

For larger tears in the small bowel, it is usually preferable to convert a longitudinal tear to a horizontal tear perpendicular to the axis of the bowel (Figure 5.12). A two-layer closure can be used. We prefer the modified one-layer Gambee closure as described below. Longitudinal lacerations of the colon may be repaired in the longitudinal plane since compromise of the lumen is unlikely. The key to the Gambee inverting suture is that the knots are on the inside. Any pelvic surgeon should be able to use simple repairs. All lacerations should be repaired as soon as they are recognized.

"Unrecognized" Injuries

Diagnosis

In the absence of acute signs, most bowel injuries present as enterovaginal or enterocutaneous fistulas. These are associated with fairly typical signs of foul drainage, sometimes interpreted by the surgeon as a "deep stitch abscess."

With persistent drainage, whether through the vagina or skin, some simple diagnostic tests are helpful. Patients can ingest charcoal, congo red dye, carmine dye, or Povan. Appearance of one of these materials at the drainage site confirms the diagnosis of bowel fistula. A fistulogram usually pinpoints the origin. A barium enema may be helpful in selected cases. Milk or methylene blue dye inserted into the rectum may help identify small rectovaginal fistulas. For complex fistulas, other studies may be necessary.

Timing of Repair

Many "unrecognized" bowel injuries result in fistulas. In the absence of acute abdominal signs, there is no need to rush to repair most gastrointestinal fistulas. Obviously, more proximal small bowel fistulas resulting in electrolyte imbalance can lead to significant morbidity and mortality. These fistulas are rarely seen in gynecologic-associated surgery.

Spontaneous closure of both small and large bowel fistulas has been reported in over 50% of nonirradiated patients when they were managed with bowel rest and total parental nutrition.[55] Even elemental diets have led to spontaneous closure of a variety of fistulas in over 50% of patients.[56] It would seem prudent to delay fistula closure in some patients for 4 to 6 weeks. However, as noted by Lichtman and McDonald,[57] some fistulas are unlikely to close with conservative measures. Such fistulas include: (1) those associated with foreign bodies, such as permanent sutures; (2) those associated with obstruction distal to the fistula; (3) those associated with epithelialization of the fistula tract; and (4) those associated with a fistula tract greater than 1 cm.

Repairing Major Injuries of Small Bowel

Fistulas usually require some type of resection or bypass. The general gynecologist is rarely required to perform a resection and reanastomosis. With an acute injury and absence of a general surgeon or gynecologic oncologist, a surgeon capable of reanastomosing a fallopian tube is capable of reuniting a vicus with a much larger lumen. Attention to detail is mandatory. Bowel contents should be suctioned from the injury site and the injured segment brought into the wound with appropriate isolation with lap pads. Rubber-shod clamps on the proximal and distal viable bowel will help avoid spillage.

The single-layer Gambee open technique is preferred over the traditional two-layer closure. It has the advantage of being faster and technically easier than the two-layered closure. All sutures can be placed under direct vision. It does not compromise the blood supply, and the lumen is less likely to be compromised. It is of particular value when used to repair previously irradiated bowel.[58-60]

In resecting loops of small bowel, only a small amount of mesentery must be removed. Hemostasis of ligated mesenteric vessels must be meticulously maintained. The open anastomosis begins with a mesenteric border suture of 3-0 polypropylene or silk. This bite should include serosa-muscularis and muscularis-serosa (Figure 5.13). Interrupted sutures of 3-0 polyglycolic acid are started at the mesenteric border and carried out to each corner and include *all* layers. This is a mucosa-muscularis-serosa to serosa-muscularis-mucosa placement (Figure 5.14). Sutures should not be tied too tightly to avoid strangulation of viable tissue. The "corner" sutures are placed in a similar manner so the knot will be on the inside (Figure 5.15). When the middle is reached from each end on the antimesenteric border, a Gambee far-near-near-far inverting suture

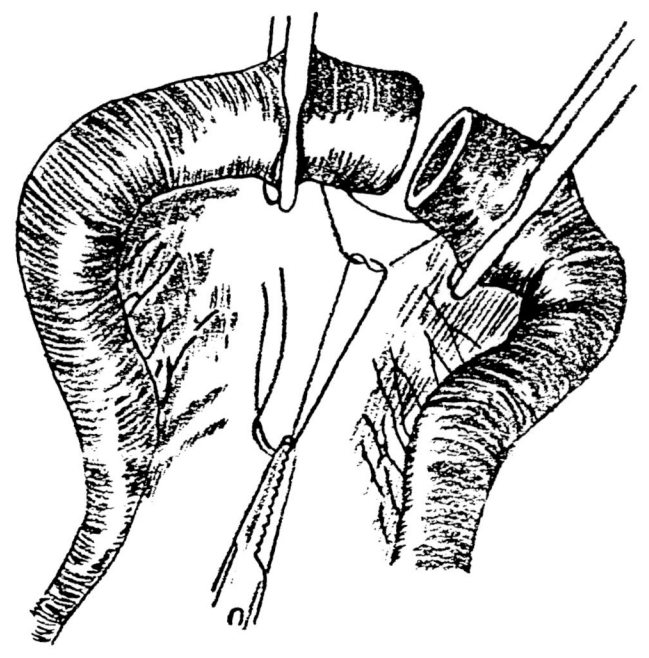

Figure 5.13 The Gambee closure. A permanent suture is placed about 5 mm from the edge on the mesenteric side.

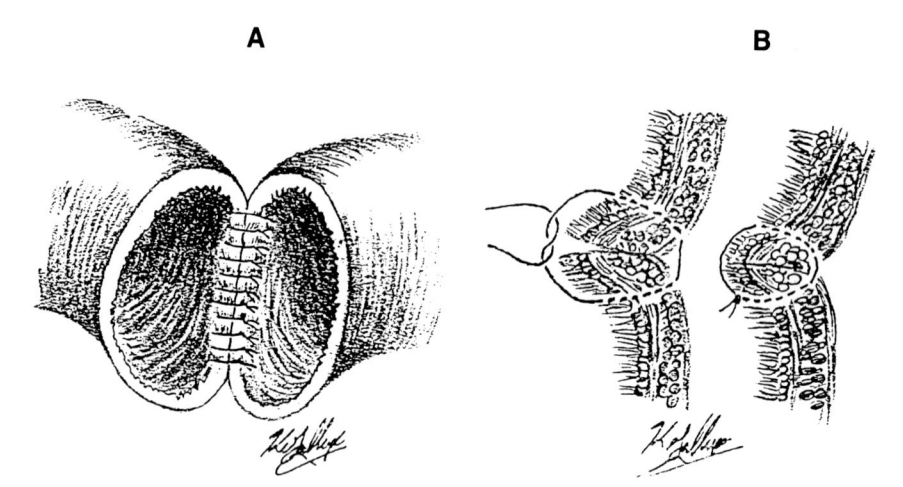

Figure 5.14 The Gambee closure. Sutures have been placed about 3 mm from the edge and 5 mm apart to close the posterior wall **(A)**. This is a through-and-through technique, and the knot is tied on the inside of the lumen **(B)**.

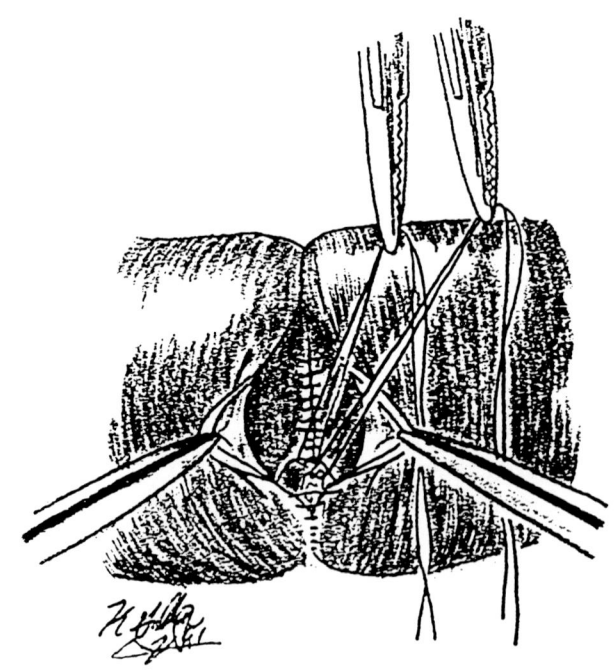

Figure 5.15 The Gambee closure. "Corner" sutures are placed so the knot is on the inside. Holding the previous suture until the next is tied will help invert the tissues.

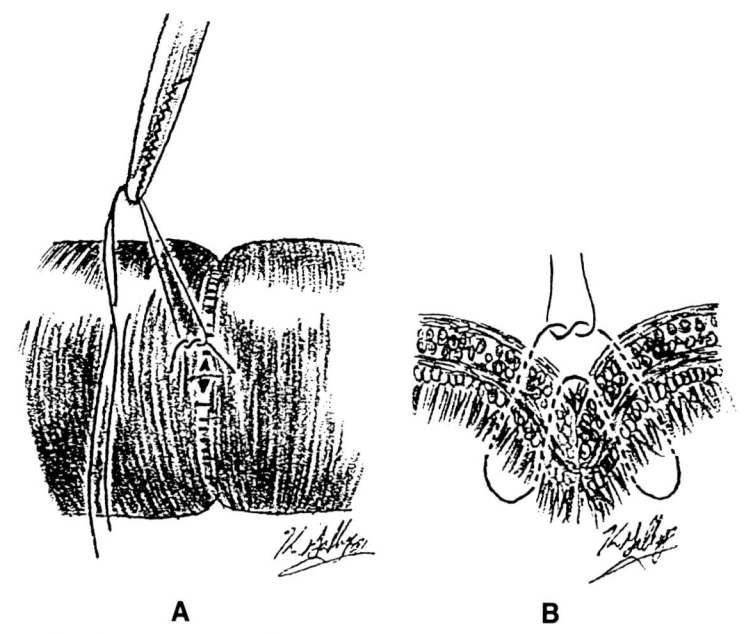

Figure 5.16 The Gambee closure. The middle has been reached, and an inverting "Gambee" suture placed at the antimesenteric border **(A)**. This is a far (5 mm)–near (3 mm)–near-far suture **(B)**.

is used (Figure 5.16). Tension-relieving serosal sutures are placed at the lateral borders (Figure 5.17), and the lumen is checked for patency. When closing the abdomen, one must always ensure that the repaired bowel is not near the anterior abdominal wall.

An alternative to the Gambee technique is using stapling instruments, which makes closure even more rapid. Lumens are less compromised than with manual techniques. The blood supply is less compromised. The tissue is handled less, and healing may be quicker because there is relatively less edema. Many gynecologic oncologists prefer staples to manual closure and report excellent results, even in presence of irradiated bowel.[61-63] Since surgical stapling instruments are not always available and the general gynecologist may be unfamiliar with their use, the surgeon may more easily rely on the Gambee single-layer closure.

Repairing Large Bowel Injuries

Large bowel injuries may be divided into those below the peritoneal reflection and those above the peritoneal reflection. For injuries below the peritoneal reflection, a one-layer Gambee closure or a two-layer closure can be utilized. For small lacerations above the peritoneal reflection, a one- or two-layer closure can be used. As with all bowel injuries, the area must be irrigated with copious amounts (at least 5 L) of Ringer's lactate. We prefer to insert a retroperitoneal drain deep in the pelvis with

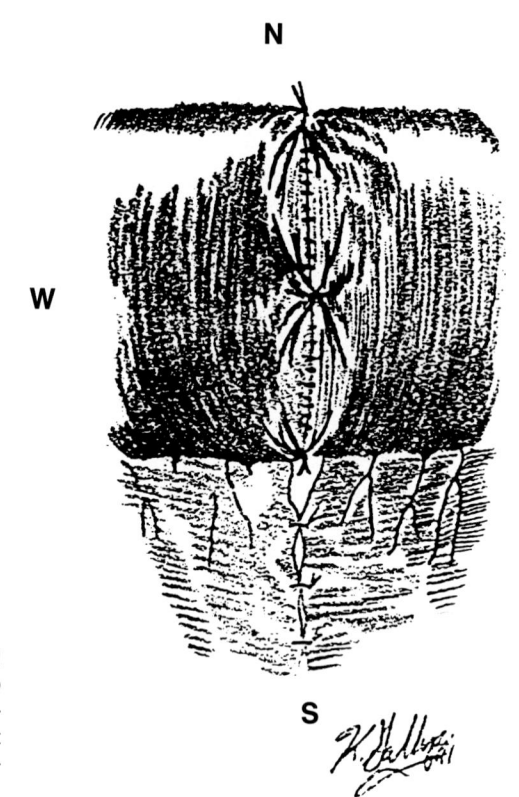

Figure 5.17 The Gambee closure. **N** (north) is the antimesenteric border. Two tension-relieving sutures of 3-0 polypropylene are placed at the east **(E)** and west **(W)** positions 5 mm from the edge and include the serosa and muscularis.

low-lying injuries. Large colon lacerations above the peritoneal reflection or lacerations associated with prior irradiation or diverticulitis may occasionally require a temporary diverting colostomy following repair. This colostomy can be closed secondarily in 6 to 8 weeks. Suspected small rectal/sigmoid injuries can be identified intraoperatively by filling the pelvis with saline and milking the descending colon. The appearance of bubbles is diagnostic.

A diverting (usually temporary) transverse loop colostomy is a relatively simple procedure that can be done by any gynecologist when general surgical or gynecologic oncology consultation is occasionally unavailable. The transverse colon can be easily recognized by its haustral markings and its attachment to the omentum. After dissection of omental and fatty tags from the colon, an avascular space (preferably in the more distal portion) of the transverse mesocolon is located. A Penrose drain is brought through the avascular space and the colon brought through the upper part of a vertical incision or through a separate small transverse upper abdominal incision.

Many new plastic products are available that have replaced the "glass rod." Any of these plastic devices can be inserted into the avascular space. Once the abdominal incision is closed with a plastic rod or Hollister bridge in the avascular space, we prefer to mature the colostomy in the operating room. The colon is incised (preferably along the tenia) in its longitudinal axis with a Bovie knife. The edges of the colon are sutured to the skin with several interrupted sutures of 3-0 polygycolic acid.

References

1. Lee RA, Symmonds RE, Williams TJ: Current status of genitourinary fistula. *Obstet Gynecol* 1988;71:313–319.
2. Symmonds RE: Incontinence: Vesical and urethral fistulas. *Clin Obstet Gynecol* 1984;27:499–514.
3. Mattingly RF, Thompson JD: Vesicovaginal fistulas, in Mattingly RF, Thompson JD (eds): *TeLinde's Operative Gynecology,* ed 6. New York, JB Lippincott Co, 1985, pp. 637–667.
4. Harrison KA: Obstetric fistula: One social calamity too many. *Br J Obstet Gynaecol* 1983;90:385–386.
5. Tahzib F: Epidemiological determinants of vesicovaginal fistulas. *Br J Obstet Gynaecol* 1983;90:387–391.
6. Murphy M: Social consequences of vesicovaginal fistula in northern Nigeria. *J Biosoc Sci* 1981;13:139–150.
7. Moir C: Vesicovaginal fistula. Thoughts on treatment of 350 cases. *Proc R Soc Med* 1966;59:1019–1022.
8. Collins CG, Jones FB: Preoperative cortisone for vaginal fistulas. *Obstet Gynecol* 1957;9:533–537.
9. Collins CG, Collins JH, Harrison BR, et al: Early repair of vesicovaginal fistula. *Am J Obstet Gynecol* 1971;111:524–528.
10. Goodwin WE, Scardino PT: Vesicovaginal and ureterovaginal fistulas: A summary of 25 years of experience. *J Urol* 1980;123:370–374.
11. Persky L, Herman G, Guerrier K: Nondelay in vesicovaginal fistula repair. *Urology* 1979;13:273–275.
12. Fearl CL, Keizur LW: Optimum time interval from occurrence to repair of vesicovaginal fistula. *Am J Obstet Gynecol* 1969;104:205–208.
13. Taylor JS, Hewson AD, Rachow P, et al: Synchronous combined transvaginal-transvesical repair of vesicovaginal fistulas. *Aust N Z J Surg* 1980;50:23–25.
14. Latzko W: Postoperative vesicovaginal fistulas: Genesis and therapy. *Am J Surg* 1942;58:211–228.
15. Keettel WC, Sehring FG, Prosse CA, et al: Surgical management of urethrovaginal and vesicovaginal fistulas. *Am J Obstet Gynecol* 1978;131:425–431.
16. Marshall VF: Vesicovaginal fistulas on one urological service. *J Urol* 1979; 121:25–29.
17. Tancer ML: The post-total hysterectomy (vault) vesicovaginal fistulas. *J Urol* 1980;123:839–840.
18. Gallup DG, Talledo OE: Diagnosis and management of the patient with a fistula, in Phelan JP, Clark SL (eds): *Cesarean Delivery.* New York, Elsevier Science Publishing Co, 1988, pp 449–461.
19. Lawson JB: The management of genito-urinary fistulae. *Clin Obstet Gynecol* 1978;5:209–236.

20. Clegg DR: Vaginal repair of obstetric vesicovaginal fistulae. *Cent Afr J Med* 1979;25:67–71.
21. Eklins TE, Drescher C, Martey JO, et al: Vesicovaginal fistula revisited. *Obstet Gynecol* 1988;72:307–312.
22. Mengert WF: Vesicovaginal fistula: Principles of closure. *Am J Obstet Gynecol* 1962;84:1213–1221.
23. Zimmern PE, Hadley HR, Staskin DR, et al: Genitourinary fistulae. Vaginal approach for repair of vesicovaginal fistulae. *Urol Clin North Am* 1985;12:361–367.
24. Martius: *Gynecological Operations: With Emphasis on Topographic Anatomy,* McCall ML, Bolten KA (trans-eds). Boston, Little, Brown, & Company, 1957, p 322.
25. Boronow RC: Repair of the radiation-induced vaginal fistula utilizing the Martius technique. *World J Surg* 1986;10:237–248.
26. Betson JR: The bulbocavernous fat pad transplant for severe stress incontinence and vesicovaginal fistula: Rationale of the procedure, indications and technique. *Am Surg* 1961;27:129–136.
27. Elkins TE, DeLancey JOL, McGuire EJ: The use of modified Martius graft as an adjunctive technique in vesicovaginal and rectovaginal fistula repair. *Obstet Gynecol* 1990;75:727–733.
28. Hoskins WJ, Park RC, Long R, et al: Repair of urinary tract fistulas with bulbocavernous myocutaneous flaps. *Obstet Gynecol* 1984;63:588–593.
29. O'Conor VJ Jr: Review of experience with vesicovaginal fistula repair. *J Urol* 1980;123:367–369.
30. Zinman LM, Libertino JA, Roth RA: Management of operative ureteral injury. *Urology* 1978;12:290–303.
31. Halloway HJ: Injury to the urinary tract as a complication of gynecologic surgery. *Am J Obstet Gynecol* 1950;60:30–40.
32. Mann WJ, Arato M, Pastner B, et al: Ureteral injuries in an obstetric and gynecology training program: Etiology and management. *Obstet Gynecol* 1988;72:82–85.
33. Cruikshank SH: Surgical method of identifying the ureters during total vaginal hysterectomy. *Obstet Gynecol* 1986;67:277–280.
34. Timmons MC, Addison WA: Suprapubic teloscopy: Extraperitoneal intraoperative technique to demonstrate ureteral patency. *Obstet Gynecol* 1990;75:137–139.
35. Hoch WH, Kursh ED, Persky L: Early aggressive management of intraoperative ureteral injuries. *J Urol* 1975;114:530–532.
36. Beland G: Early treatment of ureteral injuries found after gynecologic surgery. *J Urol* 1977;118:25–27.
37. Blandy JP, Anderson JD: Management of the injured ureter. *Proc R Soc Med* 1977;70:187–188.
38. Tarkington MA, Dejter SW Jr, Bresette JF: Early surgical management of extensive gynecologic ureteral injuries. *Surgery* 1991;173:17–21.
39. Ho PC, Talner LB, Parsons CL, et al: Percutaneous nephrostomy: Experience in 107 kidneys. *Urology* 1980;16:532–535.
40. Lang EK, Lanasa JA, Garrett J, et al: The management of urinary fistulas and strictures with percutaneous stent catheters. *J Urol* 1979;122:736–740.
41. Fisher HA, Bennett AH, Rivard DJ, et al: Nonoperative supravesical urinary diversion in obstetrics and gynecology. *Gynecol Oncol* 1982;14:365–372.

42. Hulse CA, Sawtelle WW, Nadig PW, et al: Conservative management of ureterovaginal fistula. *J Urol* 1968;99:42–49.
43. Pettit PD: Double-J ureteral catheters in gynecologic surgery. *Obstet Gynecol* 1989;73:536–540.
44. Lang EK: Diagnosis and management of ureteral fistula by percutaneous nephrostomy and antegrade stent catheter. *Radiology* 1981;138:311–317.
45. Symmonds RE: Ureteral injuries associated with gynecologic surgery: Prevention and management. *Clin Obstet Gynecol* 1976;19:623–644.
46. Politano VAW, Leadbetter WF: An operative technique for the correction of vesicoureteral reflux. *J Urol* 1958;79:932–941.
47. Thompson IM, Ross G Jr: Long-term results of bladder flap repair of ureteral injuries. *J Urol* 1974;111:483–487.
48. Lee RA, Symmonds RE: Ureterovaginal fistula. *Am J Obstet Gynecol* 1971;109:1032–1035.
49. Wheeless CR: Ureteroneocystostomy associated with gynecologic malignancy—to tunnel or not to tunnel. Presented at the Society of Gynecologic Oncologists, Palm Springs, CA, Feb 4, 1986.
50. Harrow BR: A neglected maneuver for ureterovesical implantation following injury at gynecological operations. *J Urol* 1968;100:280–287.
51. Ockerblad NE: Reimplantation of the ureter into the bladder by a flap method. *J Urol* 1947;57:845–847.
52. Demel R: Plastic reconstruction of ureter from bladder. *Zentralbl Chir* 1924;51:2008–2011.
53. Fry DE, Milholen L, Harbrecht PJ: Iatrogenic ureteral injury. Options in management. *Arch Surg* 1983;118:454–457.
54. Beland G: The abdominal surgeon and the ureter. *Can J Surg* 1979;22:540–541,544.
55. Hew LR, Deitel M: Total parenteral nutrition in gynecology and obstetrics. *Obstet Gynecol* 1980;55:464–468.
56. Bury KD, Stephens RV, Randall HT: Use of a chemically defined liquid, elemental diet for nutritional management of fistulas of the alimentary tract. *Am J Surg* 1971;121:174–183.
57. Lichtman AL, McDonald JR: Fecal fistula. *Surg Gynecol Obstet* 1944;78:449–470.
58. Gambee LP, Garnjobst W, Hardwick CE: Ten years' experience with a single layer anastomosis in colon surgery. *Am J Surg* 1956;92:222–227.
59. Wheeless CR: The Gambee intestinal anastomosis in gynecologic surgery. *Obstet Gynecol* 1975;46:448–452.
60. Miholic J, Schlappack O, Kleptko W, et al: Surgical therapy of radiation-induced small-bowel injuries. *Arch Surg* 1987;122:923–926.
61. Wheeless CR: Stapling techniques in operations for malignant disease of the female genital tract. *Surg Clin North Am* 1984;64:591–608.
62. Rubin SC, Benjamin I, Hoskins WJ, et al: Intestinal surgery in gynecologic oncology. *Gynecol Oncol* 1989;34:30–33.
63. Barnhill D, Doering D, Remmenga S, et al: Intestinal surgery performed on gynecologic cancer patients. *Gynecol Oncol* 1991;40:38–41.

Chapter 6

Management of Intraoperative and Postoperative Hemorrhage at the Time of Hysterectomy

James L. Breen, MD, and John T. Comerci, MD

Regardless of how well planned and skillfully executed, every gynecologic procedure is characterized by a certain irreducible loss of blood that is directly related to the magnitude of the operation, the vascularity of the surgical field, and the knowledge and experience of the surgeon. In the majority of gynecologic surgical procedures, slow anatomic dissection coupled with the application of the basic principles of hemostasis will keep blood loss to an acceptable minimum. The surgeon's goal should be to anticipate and prevent hemorrhage rather than struggle to halt it when it occurs. This chapter focuses on techniques to prevent hemorrhage and also outlines management schemes regarding intra- and postoperative bleeding.

Categories of Surgical Bleeding

Intraoperative bleeding may be characterized by either injury to specific blood vessels or bleeding secondary to defects in the normal clotting mechanism. The former type of bleeding relates to the skill of the surgeon as well as the nature of the surgery being performed, and usually responds to direct compression or ligation of the injured vessel. The latter is characterized by a persistent oozing of blood from operative sites and requires correction of the coagulation defect by platelet component and plasma replacement. The inability to surgically control bleeding may lead to a bleeding diathesis from platelet washout and a decrease in coagulation components secondary to massive transfusion.

Defects of the Clotting Mechanism

Defects of the clotting mechanism can be most easily understood if the hemostatic mechanism is divided into its basic components: vascular,

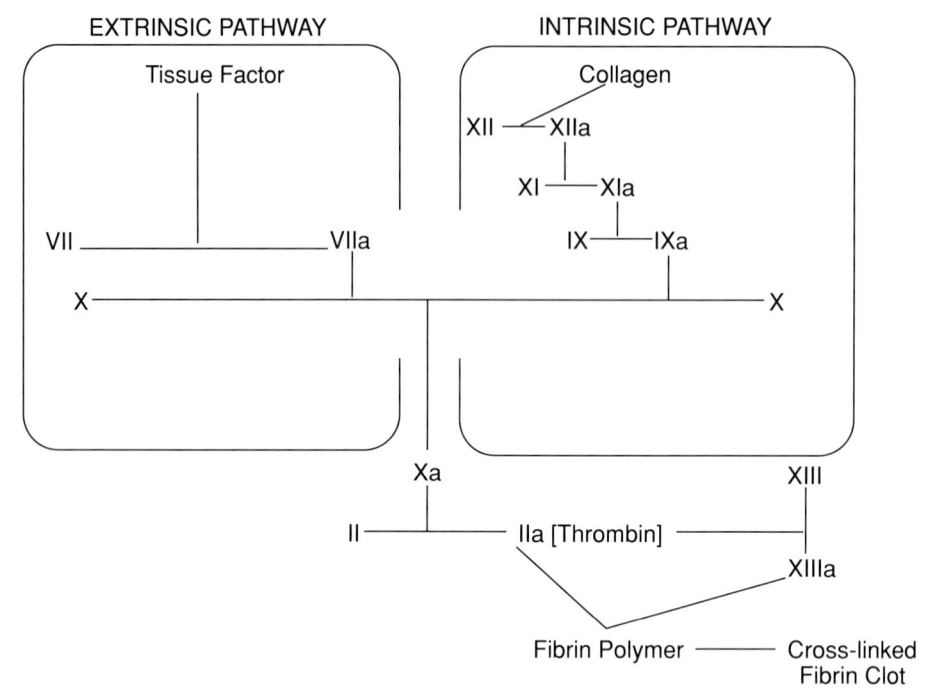

Figure 6.1 Outline of intrinsic and extrinsic coagulation systems. Both extrinsic and intrinsic systems converge to activate Factor X.

formed elements, and plasma coagulation factors. Alteration in one or more of these components can result in a bleeding diathesis.

When the integrity of a blood vessel wall is breached, underlying collagen, microfibrils, and the basement membrane are exposed. Platelets adhere to the wound site and become activated. Platelet activation entails the release of thromboxane, which causes platelet aggregation and vasoconstriction.[1,2] Vascular injury produces a tissue factor that initiates the extrinsic pathway by activating factor VII to VIIa. Factor VIIa in turn activates factor X to Xa, generating factor IIa (thrombin). Thrombin feeds back to activate factors V and VII, thus further amplifying the system.[3] These mechanisms come together to form a hemostatic plug and, along with injury-induced vessel constriction, reduce the size of the vascular defect[3] (Figure 6.1).

Bleeding disorders encountered intraoperatively are either acquired or congenital.

Acquired Bleeding Disorders

Disseminated Intravascular Coagulation

Disseminated intravascular coagulation (DIC) is a disease in which platelets and fibrinogen are consumed.[4] The depletion of coagulation factors is not clinically evident until it is severe enough to cause generalized bleeding. The pathogenesis of DIC involves massive activation of hemostatic mechanisms resulting in thrombin formation. Secondarily, fibrin and fibrinogen are degraded by the fibrinolytic system.[5] It is the depletion of procoagulants and platelets that causes hemorrhage. The massive production of thrombin, in contrast, causes thrombosis in the arteriovenous systems, leading to tissue ischemia, infarction, and necrosis. Tissue necrosis in turn causes increased tissue activation of the hemostatic system and thus increased consumption of coagulation factors.

These thrombotic events affect all organ systems. The skin may manifest patchy necrosis.[6] The renal system may fail secondary to destruction of the glomerular capillaries, causing hematuria, oligemia, or anuria.[7] Finally, pulmonary capillary destruction can lead to interstitial hemorrhage, causing hypoxemia and the adult respiratory distress syndrome.[8]

Disseminated intravascular coagulation may have a number of initiating factors, including tissue damage, either traumatic or obstetric; shock secondary to hypovolemia; neoplasia; and gram-negative sepsis. All have the same effect—the production of thrombin and the massive consumption of procoagulants and platelets. Management must be directed at eliminating the causative events while applying supportive measures.

Bleeding Secondary to Transfusion

Intraoperative hemorrhage may be directly related to blood transfusions either from a transfusion reaction in which an antigen-antibody reaction causes hemolysis, and DIC,[9] or dilution of coagulation factors as a result of deficiencies of factors V, VII, and XI in stored blood.[10,11] The most common cause of bleeding associated with massive transfusion is thrombocytopenia secondary to platelet washout and platelet dysfunction.[12] The qualitative platelet abnormality may be secondary to either mechanical damage or coating of the platelets with fibrin degradation products that inhibit their aggregation. Functional platelets are not present in stored blood, so platelet transfusions are paramount in patients who received massive transfusions but continue to bleed.

Hypothermia (defined as a core temperature of 32°C or less) is commonly encountered in a patient undergoing massive transfusions and may impair the coagulation mechanism. Efforts to warm blood should be made during massive transfusion because the coagulation system is enzymatic and functions best in physiologic temperature ranges. Although the quantity of coagulation factors does not fall during hypothermia, their activity is depressed.[13] In addition, hypothermia impairs the metabolism of citrate and lactate, thus increasing hypocalcemia and metabolic acidosis. It also increases the affinity of hemoglobin for oxygen, and impairs red cell deformity.[14] Valeri et al[15] demonstrated a decreased platelet activity, as measured by the production of thromboxane B_2, in hypothermic baboons.

Acquired Procoagulant Disorders

Other acquired disorders of coagulation include decreased synthesis of coagulation factors secondary to liver disease, drug-induced hemorrhage resulting from treatment with heparin or warfarin, dysproteinemias such as myeloma and macroglobulinemia, and the presence of circulating anticoagulants such as the lupus anticoagulant factor.[3]

Acquired Platelet Disorders

A frequently encountered coagulation defect in surgical patients is a functional platelet defect caused by drug ingestion. Characteristically, functional platelet disorders cause a prolonged bleeding time despite a normal platelet count. Aspirin and other nonsteroidal antiinflammatory medications, such as indomethacin, phenylbutazone, and ibuprofen, are responsible for most cases of drug-induced platelet dysfunction.

Aspirin irreversibly acetylates cyclooxygenase in platelets and blocks the synthesis of thromboxane A_2. The effect lasts the lifetime of the platelets (approximately 7 to 10 days) and will continue until new platelets overcome the antiplatelet effect.[5]

Antibiotics are another class of drugs that cause acquired functional platelet disorders. Carbenicillin and ticarcillin[16] as well as moxalactam, a third-generation cepholosporin,[17] can inhibit platelet aggregation. If an antibiotic-related bleeding disorder is suspected, antibiotics should be withdrawn or the dosage reduced. Because their effects may be additive, simultaneous use of these antibiotics and nonsteroidal antiinflammatory agents should be avoided. Systemic diseases such as uremia, myloproliferative disorders, idiopathic thrombocytopenic purpura, and liver disease may also be responsible for qualitative platelet dysfunction.

Congenital Bleeding Disorders

Congenital Procoagulant Disorders

Inherited coagulation disorders such as hemophilia and von Willebrand's disease occur in approximately 1 in 10,000 people.[5] Hemophilia A is a deficiency of factor VIIIc.[18] It is a sex-linked recessive disorder in which 20% of affected patients have a negative family history.[19] Hemophilia B (Christmas disease) is caused by a deficiency in factor IX and occurs less frequently than hemophilia A. Clinically hemophilia A and B are indistinguishable.[5] Von Willebrand's disease is a mild bleeding disorder that is caused by an abnormality of factor VIII complex that is different from the abnormality causing hemophilia A.[20]

Congenital Platelet Disorders

Hereditary quantitative platelet disorders are divided into defective platelet production, such as hereditary thrombocytopenia, and increased platelet destruction, such as the Wiskott-Aldrich syndrome.[21] Platelet defects of adhesion (Benard-Soulier syndrome), primary aggregation (thromboasthenia), and secretion (storage pool disease) have all been described.[22]

Preoperative Diagnosis of a Bleeding Diathesis

Paramount in diagnosing a bleeding diathesis preoperatively are the history and physical examination. Pertinent questions include bleeding problems associated with previous surgery, either major or minor (tooth extractions); family history of bleeding problems; gingival bleeding secondary to dental hygiene; spontaneous bleeding into muscles, joints, and subcutaneous tissue; tendency to bruise easily; recent or prolonged drug ingestion (eg, aspirin, warfarin); and frequent or recurrent epistaxis and hematuria. Pertinent physical signs and symptoms generally make it possible to diagnose disorders of the coagulating system preoperatively. Mild coagulation defects, however, may be unsuspected if the patient has not been previously traumatized or subjected to major or minor surgical procedures.

Laboratory tests routinely utilized as a preoperative screening procedure include complete blood count, prothrombin test, partial thromboplastin time test, and inspection of the blood smear to determine platelet adequacy. When additional investigations are warranted, it is advisable to determine platelet counts, bleeding and clotting times, clot retraction, and fibrinogen levels. If the extrinsic and intrinsic clotting systems are normal (as reflected by a normal prothrombin test and partial thromboplastin time test) and if platelets are adequate, but the patient manifests signs or symptoms of a bleeding diathesis, a qualitative platelet defect must be considered. The salient features of qualitative platelet abnormalities are bleeding with lacerations or surgery, lack of petechiae, increased platelet counts, and a prolonged bleeding time.

Intraoperative Bleeding
Initial Assessment and Management of Bleeding Diatheses

Even though the possibility of a preexisting bleeding diathesis has been explored, it should be remembered that defects in the normal hemostatic process may develop intraoperatively. Generalized oozing may develop during a surgical procedure even after good initial hemostasis.

The amount and rate of bleeding determine the signs and symptoms of hemorrhage. A loss of up to 15% of the circulating blood volume may not necessarily cause changes in blood or pulse pressure. A systemic hemorrhagic disorder is characterized by bleeding at multiple sites (eg, around a catheter and from venipuncture sites). Initial assessment requires a hematocrit, platelet count, prothrombin test, and partial thromboplastin time test.

Patients who respond to 3 L of crystalloid solution have usually lost less than 50% of their circulating blood volume and will not need additional replacement therapy. Coagulation factors and platelets are present in much greater concentrations than are usually needed for hemostasis. For example, factor VIII levels may fall as low as 30% of normal before normal clotting is affected.[5] Patients who do not respond to crystalloid solution have usually lost greater than 50% of their circulating blood volume and should initially receive two units of packed cells.[5]

Many replacement formulas have been advocated for the treatment of excessive hemorrhage.[23–28] A frequently proposed formula is the addition of one unit of fresh frozen plasma and one ampule of calcium chloride for every four to five units of packed red blood cells.[29] The empiric use of fresh frozen plasma has been the subject of much debate. No correlation between the prothrombin test/partial thromboplastin time test and units of fresh frozen plasma and packed red blood cells has been found.[30] In fact, microvascular bleeding secondary to massive hemorrhage has been found to be more closely correlated to thrombocytopenia (platelet count less than 50,000) and hypofibrinogenemia (defined as less than 0.5 mg/dL) than clotting factor dilution. Hence the use of platelets and fibrinogen in the form of cryoprecipitate may be more efficacious than fresh frozen plasma. A unit of platelets contains between 5,500 and 8,000 platelets and will increase the circulating platelet count by this amount.[31] In most institutions, platelets are supplied in six- to ten-unit packs. Cryoprecipitate contains factor VIII and von Willebrand factor, fibronectin, and fibrinogen. Each unit contains 80 units of factor VIII and 200 mg fibrinogen.[32]

Generally, the indications for the use of fresh frozen plasma include the replacement of isolated deficiencies (most commonly of factors II, V, VII, X, and XI), the reversal of warfarin in emergency surgery, massive transfusion (greater than total blood volume in several hours or approximately ten units packed red blood cells), and treatment of humoral immunodeficiencies.[33] The use of platelets is effective in controlling generalized oozing from the surgical site after adequate hemostasis has been obtained. If there is ongoing hemorrhage with the expectation of continued loss, platelet counts greater than 50,000 should be maintained.[32] Finally, the patient with an intraoperative bleeding diathesis with fibrinogen levels less than 50 to 100 mg/dL should be considered for treatment with cryoprecipitate (0.1 to 0.15 units/kg of body weight).[32] It should be noted that acquiring these blood products takes time, and their potential use must be anticipated if an intraoperative bleeding diathesis is to be reversed.

Anatomy and Physiology of Pelvic Bleeding

Familiarity with the vascular anatomy of the pelvis is imperative in the performance of pelvic surgery and in the control of intraoperative hemorrhage. There is a complex primary and collateral circulation to pelvic

Table 6.1 Divisions of the Hypogastric Artery

Posterior Division	Anterior Division	
Parietal Branches	Parietal Branches	Visceral Branches
Iliolumbar	Obturator	Umbilical
Lateral sacral	Internal pudendal	Uterine
Superior gluteal	Inferior gluteal	Vaginal
		Superior vesical
		Inferior vesical
		Middle hemorrhoidal

organs. The major blood supply is provided by branches of the anterior division of the internal iliac (hypogastric) artery (Table 6.1). The hypogastric artery originates at the bifurcation of the common iliac artery, opposite to the lumbosacral intervertebral disc and in front of the sacroiliac joint. It then descends to the upper part of the greater sciatic foramen, dividing into the anterior and posterior trunks. The latter gives off the iliolumbar and lateral sacral arteries before leaving the pelvis via the greater sciatic foramen as the superior gluteal artery. The obturator, superior vesicle, inferior vesicle, uterine, vaginal, middle hemorrhoidal, inferior hemorrhoidal, and pudendal arteries are derived from the anterior trunk.

A simple equation can be employed to determine the rate of blood loss from injured or unligated blood vessels:

$$\dot{Q} = S \sqrt{\frac{P_I - P_E}{e} + V^2}$$

In this equation, $\dot{Q}$ is the rate of blood loss, S is the surface area of the laceration, P_E is the extravascular pressure, P_I is the intravascular pressure, e is the density of the blood, and V is the velocity of blood flow in the vessel. A suture that reduces S to 0 will cease all blood flow. Ligation of the hypogastric artery will reduce flow by decreasing both V and P_I. Of course, the patient in shock will have low P_I and V values and may present a problem to the surgeon trying to identify the injured vessel during extreme hypotensive periods, which explains the occasional need for reexploration. This formula does not, however, take into account the status of the patient's coagulation system.

Prevention

Although intraoperative hemorrhage may occur in any patient, despite the most careful surgical techniques, its stage is usually set by an inappropriate abdominal incision, speed or impatience on the part of the surgeon, improper handling of tissues, or poor surgical technique.

Exposure

The most important factor in the prevention and control of unexpected intraoperative hemorrhage is proper and adequate exposure. Several factors are important in obtaining adequate exposure. These include the type of incision utilized, able surgical assistance, correct type and number of surgical retractors, good operating room lighting, and proper anesthesia.

If there is any question concerning the exposure needed for the procedure, a vertical midline incision provides the greatest exposure and should be the incision of choice. Individual Deaver retractors allow more diversity and individuality with regard to exposing different areas of the operative field and are preferable to a stationary field with self-retaining retractors. The bowel should be kept out of the operative field by placing the patient in a Trendelenburg position. A hand should be placed in the pelvis with the palmer surface up. Three laparotomy pads should be rolled off the palm into the abdomen, first in the midline and then to the right and left sides, thus packing the bowel away from the operative field. In extreme emergencies the surgeon should not pack the bowel, but instead eviscerate the patient and hold the bowel with wet laps on the anterior abdominal wall.

Surgical Technique

Regarding the role of proper surgical technique in the prevention of surgical bleeding, several points may be considered; (1) sharp rather than blunt dissection, (2) identification and isolation of vascular pedicles, (3) proper utilization of vascular and pedicle clamps, (4) avoidance of mass ligatures, (5) single versus double ligation of vascular pedicles, and (6) care in handling ligated vascular pedicles.

By avoiding blunt tissue dissection with gauze pads or gauze within sponge loops, generalized oozing from sheared blood vessels is decreased. Hence, the use of sharp tissue dissection with scissors or scalpel will ultimately improve identification and decrease the devitalization and necrosis of tissues.

Where the field of dissection is altered because of a loss of landmarks or increased vascularity as a result of an inflammatory or neoplastic disease, isolating the vessels supplying the area is essential to prevent undue blood loss. For example, temporary occlusion or ligation of the internal iliac arteries or temporary occlusion of the aorta just above its bifurcation may be worthwhile.

Several specific surgical principles regarding the handling of tissue pedicles are essential to reduce the risk of intraoperative bleeding. First, it is preferable to isolate and skeletonize vascular pedicles whenever feasible to reduce tissue or vessel retraction. Also, it should be emphasized that the purchase or action point of a surgical clamp is limited to its distal third or half. Therefore, incorporating an entire pedicle or overloading the clamp to its crutch leads to slippage of the suture or rotation of the vasculature within the pedicle. Finally, the greater the amount of tissue within a clamp, the greater the amount of tissue necrosis and slough, potentially causing a higher incidence of febrile morbidity.

Regardless of the suture material or the methodology of suture ligation, the surgeon should place the needle as close to the clamp as possible. This is facilitated by rolling the clamp to expose the tissue-clamp interface and placing the needle through the pedicle riding the surface of the clamp. Single-suture ligatures on vascular as well as other pedicles are recommended. A single, properly placed ligature is adequate for the control of bleeding and also leads to less tissue necrosis and slough.

After vascular pedicles are identified, isolated, clamped, cut, and suture ligated, they should never be held or placed on traction because this will increase the risk of laceration or intimal tearing within the vessel. In the elderly, even minimal traction on vascular pedicles may lead to laceration.

Management Principles

The most common error in the control of sudden intraoperative bleeding is blind clamping in a surgical field obscured by the accumulation of blood. This is dangerous since the usual result is further tissue damage, blood loss, and damage to adjacent structures such as the ureter, bladder, and intestinal tract. To facilitate accurate clamp placement, digital compression at the site of bleeding or direct compression with a lap pad or sponge stick usually controls bleeding and allows visualization.

In most instances, arterial bleeding is easier to control than venous oozing. The cyclic spurting action from arteries permits easier identification and more precise clamping of the vessels involved. The tonsil clamp, which is tapered from its heel to its tip, allows for easy ligature placement over the arterial stump.

If bleeding from a large vessel is massive, it is often of great help to place the end of the suction tube near the opening in the vessel to expose the exact source of the bleeding. At times temporary occlusion of the aorta with a DeBakey clamp or occlusion of the common iliac arteries with a rubber-shod bulldog clamp, as well as manual compression, will allow for the identification and securing of a bleeding point.

Since venous pressure is low, bleeding from a vein can usually be controlled by applying a finger, by compressing the vessel against a firm structure, or by grasping the vessel between fingers. These steps provide the surgeon with time to collect his or her thoughts regarding what vessel has been injured and which course of dissection is necessary to ligate it.

Any vein in the pelvis may be ligated. Even if the common or external iliac veins are ligated, the edema of the ipsilateral lower extremity is usually mild and subsides with the establishment of collateral vasculature. In fact, inferior vena cava ligation has been described for intractable pelvic hemorrhage, with occasional leg pain and bilateral lower extremity edema being the only problems reported postoperatively.[34] Damage to large significant arteries (aorta, common iliac, external iliac) must be repaired, preferably with the assistance of a vascular or general surgeon if the gynecologic surgeon has not been so trained.

Venous oozing from raw surfaces, as may be encountered in a patient with massive pelvic adhesions, extensive endometriosis, multiple leiomyomas, or pelvic carcinoma, may be managed by firm, direct pressure with warm laparotomy pads for approximately 5 minutes. If bleeding persists, sutures can be placed around multiple bleeding sites. If this fails, because bleeding is from a broad surface or tissues are too friable, the application of oxidized regenerated cellulose (Oxycel, Surgicel) or microfibrillar collagen (Avitene) is effective. Microfibrillar collagen exerts its hemostatic effect by attracting platelets, which adhere to the microbibrils and trigger the formation of thrombi in the interstices of the fibrous mass.[35]

Infundibulopelvic Ligament Hematoma

Infundibulopelvic ligament hematomas are caused by retraction of the ovarian artery or vein away from the original tie. Bleeding then occurs into the retroperitoneal compartment. It is extremely difficult to single out the ovarian artery because it is surrounded by veins. The best course of action is to dissect upward, using sharp dissection, into the retroperitoneal space. The course of the ureter should be noted at all times during this dissection. Proximal to the hematoma, where the veins become of normal caliber, a Mixter clamp can be used to pass a tie around the veins. Once the hematoma is isolated, it should be evacuated and small contributing veins cauterized or clipped. If bleeding persists in spite of the steps outlined, ligation of the ovarian artery at its origin is required.

Pelvic Packs

The surgeon is occasionally faced with controlling hemorrhage from large raw surfaces, venous plexuses, or inaccessible areas within the pelvis, often with the added problem of a coagulopathy. In these instances the surgeon may employ a pack to produce a pelvic tamponade. The umbrella or mushroom pack, used for control of bleeding primarily after radical surgical procedures, was first described by Logothelopulos in 1926.[36] He demonstrated its efficacy by placing it in a patient who had a hysterectomy without vessel ligation!

The pelvic pack consists of a square, 24 in on each side, of fine mesh gauze laparotomy pad, either cotton or nylon. Fifteen to 20 yards of 2-in gauze tape or 6 yards of 4-in head-roll gauze is layered into the center of the pack, taking care to prevent any tangling that may prevent removal.

A funnel-shaped sling is then formed when the four corners of the pad are brought together. A short tail of the gauze is left free and tagged with a suture. The diagonal corners of the pack are brought over the pack and tied. This bolus of gauze is then placed in the true pelvis with the tail exiting the vagina. If bleeding points are observed near the pelvic brim, additional gauze may be necessary. A sterile "bowel bag" may be placed over the pack to prevent bowel adherence, facilitating easier removal. The pack may also be applied through the vagina and formed inside the pelvis. In this case, the pad is held in front of the vulva by the corners, and the center is pushed through the vagina into the pelvis by inserting gauze with a ring forceps. The four corners are then brought together and pulled down to seat the pack. Approximately 2 to 5 kg of traction weight is applied to the tails of the pack for 48 to 72 hours. Tension is released every 8 hours to prevent pressure necrosis of pelvic tissues. Passing the tails through a no. 80 doughnut pessary and cross-clamping the tails with a Kelly clamp after applying sufficient traction to seat the pack are satisfactory. A Foley catheter is placed in the bladder so that the bulb is above the pack. Decreased urine output after restoration of circulating volume may indicate excessive traction. Broad-spectrum antibiotics are advisable during the use of the pack. The pack may be removed the following day under analgesia. The ends are soaked in saline and hydrogen peroxide. The pack is removed vaginally regardless of the type of insertion used.

There are cases in which a more conventional packing may be appropriate, such as in a patient with broad surface bleeding or bleeding in areas inaccessible to conventional suturing or clamping. Here, the transabdominal placement of 5-in packs in the pelvis is most effective.[35] This technique involves moving the 2-in pack from right to left, placing it over the entire pelvis, and bringing it out through a stab wound in the groin. For cases of extensive bleeding, it is often necessary to employ five or six 2-in packs. In these cases, the second pack is placed over the initial pack and brought out through a separate stab wound. It is important to remember never to tie two packs together because they must be removed through the incision in the groin. If six packs are utilized, there will be six exit sites within the groin.[37] It is helpful to tag each pack with either a safety pin or a suture, so that one knows the position of the packs, bottom and top. The topmost packs will be removed on the day after surgery and the bottom packs removed 72 hours after surgery. Again, broad-spectrum antibiotics should be used during this period.

Hypogastric Artery Ligation

Once the gynecologic surgeon has exhausted the conventional methods available to control intraoperative hemorrhage, the ultimate resolution of bleeding may be accomplished by bilateral ligation of the internal iliac (hypogastric) arteries.[22] Historically, the usefulness of this procedure has

Table 6.2 Indications for Hypogastric Artery Ligation

Indication	Type
Bleeding from malignant disease	Cervical carcinoma
	Uterine carcinoma
	Rectal carcinoma
Vascular disease or injury	Gluteal aneurysm
	Internal iliac aneurysm
	Pelvic trauma
Obstetric	Placenta accreta, increta, and percreta
	Uterine rupture
	Uterine atony
Operative	Hysterectomy (vaginal, abdominal)
	Cystectomy
	Prostatectomy
	Abdominoperineal resection
	Hot knife conization of the cervix
	Cold knife conization of the cervix
	Cryosurgery of the cervix
Postoperative	Primary or secondary postoperative hemorrhage
Elective	Anticipated operative bleeding
	Teaching

been demonstrated in many areas dealing with the pelvis and its contents[38–40] (Table 6.2). From 1969 to 1990, 462 hypogastric ligations were performed in the Department of Obstetrics and Gynecology of the Saint Barnabas Medical Center.[40] Indications are listed in Table 6.3. The main indication for the procedure is for teaching. Bilateral ligation of the hypogastric arteries is an integral part of the management of massive

Table 6.3 Hypogastric Artery Ligation Indications

Procedure	No. of Patients
Radical gynecologic surgery	
Therapeutic	5
Prophylactic	35
Teaching	358
Total abdominal hysterectomy	7
Uterine rupture	6
Vaginal hysterectomy	4
Hot knife conization of the cervix	4
Cold knife conization of the cervix	3
Cryosurgery of the cervix	3
Placenta accreta	3
Utgerine atony	3
Anterio colporrhaphy	1
TOTAL	432

Data from Saint Barnabas Medical Center, Livingston, NJ, 1969–1989.

obstetric and gynecologic hemorrhage, and it is far better to learn this technique under a controlled situation, so the surgeon can be prepared if it should become necessary.

Anatomy

The hypogastric arteries have important relationships to neighboring anatomic structures. Anteromedially, the hypogastric artery is covered by peritoneum; it is a retroperitoneal structure. On the right side of the pelvis, the terminal end of the ileum and the cecum may overlie the peritoneum. Anteriorly, the ureter lies retroperitoneally (attached to the undersurface of the peritoneum) and crosses over the hypogastric artery from lateral to medial at its origin. Posterolaterally lie the external iliac vein and the obturator nerve. The internal iliac (hypogastric vein) is situated posteromedially.

Collateral Circulation

The collateral circulation of the pelvis has been the subject of discussion for at least a century. *Gray's Anatomy* describes the presence of many anastomoses.[41] These anastomoses occur in each hemipelvis, both vertically (ipsilaterally) and horizontally (across the midline). After bilateral hypogastric artery ligation, the vertical system is the most important because there is little transmission across the midline.

There are three major vertical anastomotic channels in each hemipelvis[30]:

1. Lumbar (branch of aorta) to iliolumbar
2. Middle sacral (branch of aorta) to lateral sacral
3. Superior hemorrhoidal (branch of the inferior mesenteric) to middle hemorrhoidal

Aortographic studies have shown that all of these anastomotic channels are present before ligation and are immediately functional once the ligation is performed.[42] The reason they become functional is that the superior pressure in the lumbar, middle sacral, and superior hemorrhoidal vessels reverses the direction of blood flow in their anastomotic counterparts, which branch from the hypogastric artery below the point of ligation.

Hemodynamics

Complete cessation of blood flow is not the reason for the success of hypogastric artery ligation.[43] The procedure, while decreasing the mean uterine artery pressure and blood flow by only 24% and 48%, respectively, produces its most significant physiologic effect by reducing the arterial pulse pressure by 85%. This decrease in pulse pressure eliminates the "trip hammer" effect of arterial pulsations, allowing a stable clot to form. In effect, bilateral hypogastric artery vessel ligation transforms an arterial system into a venous one in terms of hemodynamics. It should be noted that hypogastric artery ligation does not control hemorrhage from branches of the ovarian artery or from generalized venous oozing.

Surgical Technique

Hypogastric arteries may be exposed either extraperitoneally or intraperitoneally. Intraperitoneal exposure is the preferred approach for extensive intraperitoneal bleeding. The common iliac artery and its two main branches are easily palpable and visualized along the pelvic sidewall. Care should be taken to retract the ureter and its peritoneum medially during the procedure. An attempt should be made to ligate the hypogastric artery distal to its posterior division, but many times it is easier to tie the hypogastric near its origin from the common iliac artery. The origin of the division is not always obvious but generally occurs within the first 2 to 3 cm from the iliac bifurcation. Once the site for ligation has been determined, the loose areolar tissue and adventitia are dissected from the artery. To avoid injuring the hypogastric vein, use a

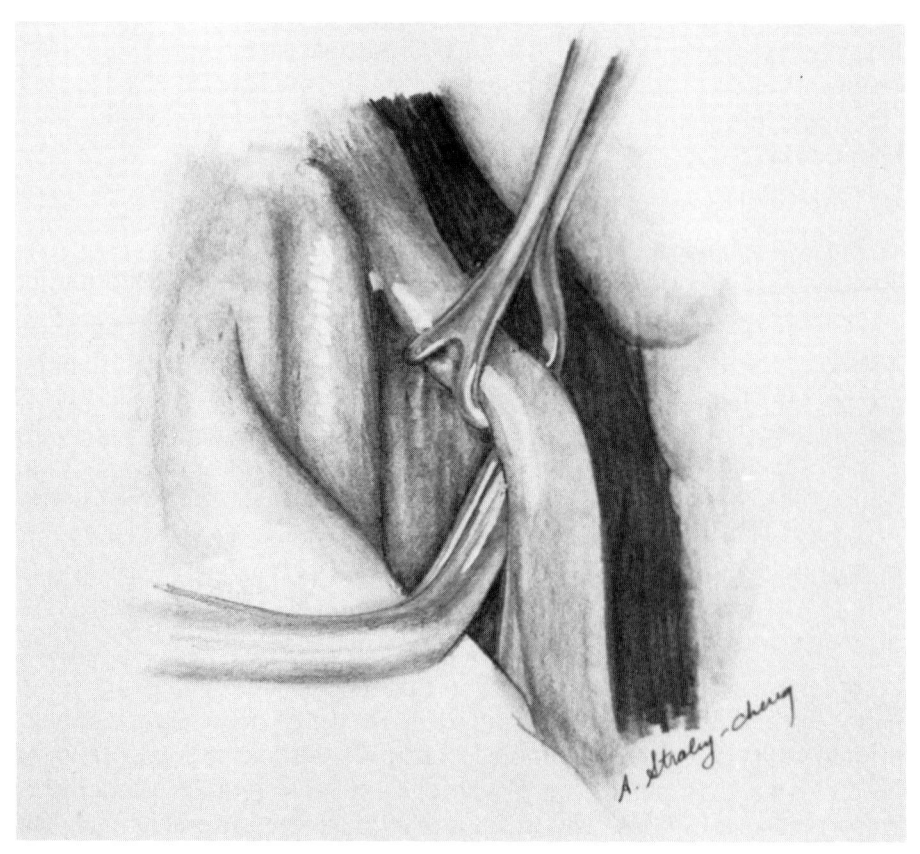

Figure 6.2 Hypogastric artery ligation. Right-angle (Mixter) clamp is being placed in areolar plane beneath the hypogastric artery, which is being elevated by a Babcock clamp.

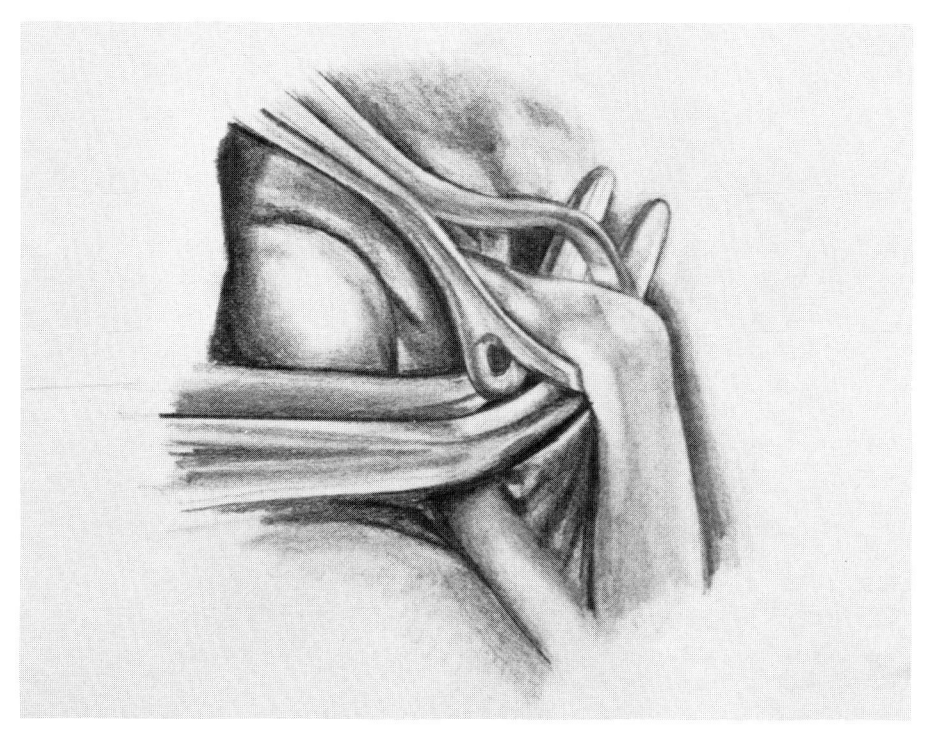

Figure 6.3 Hypogastric artery ligation. The Mixter clamp has now been opened to receive the suture.

Babcock clamp to elevate the artery. Figure 6.2 reveals a right-angle (Mixter) clamp being placed in the areolar plane beneath the hypogastric artery, which is being elevated by a Babcock clamp. The Mixter clamp is then opened to receive the suture held by an associate (Figure 6.3). The suture is placed in a tip of the Mixter clamp, thus being ready to be passed under the hypogastric artery (Figure 6.4). The suture is drawn beneath the hypogastric artery and passed to a tonsil clamp (Figure 6.5). The Mixter clamp is repositioned below the hypogastric artery and the suture on the tonsil clamp is brought down and grasped by the Mixter clamp for a "second pass" below the hypogastric artery (Figure 6.6). A double loop of suture is now in place around the hypogastric artery (Figure 6.7) and is moved to the bifurcation of the common iliac artery to be tied (Figure 6.8).

Complications and Efficacy

Technical problems associated with hypogastric artery ligation include ligating the external iliac artery or the ureter and lacerating the hypogastric vein. The surgeon should palpate the femoral pulses, identify the ureter both before and after ligation, and use extreme caution around the hypogastric vein. The major pitfall associated with ligation of the

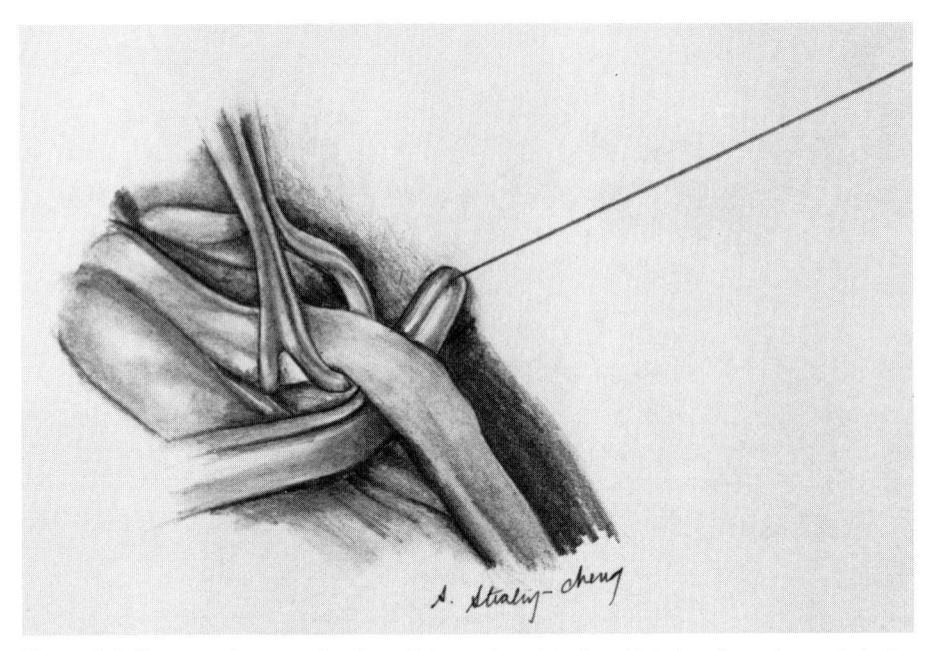

Figure 6.4 Hypogastric artery ligation. Suture placed in tip of Mixter clamp is ready to be passed under the hypogastric artery.

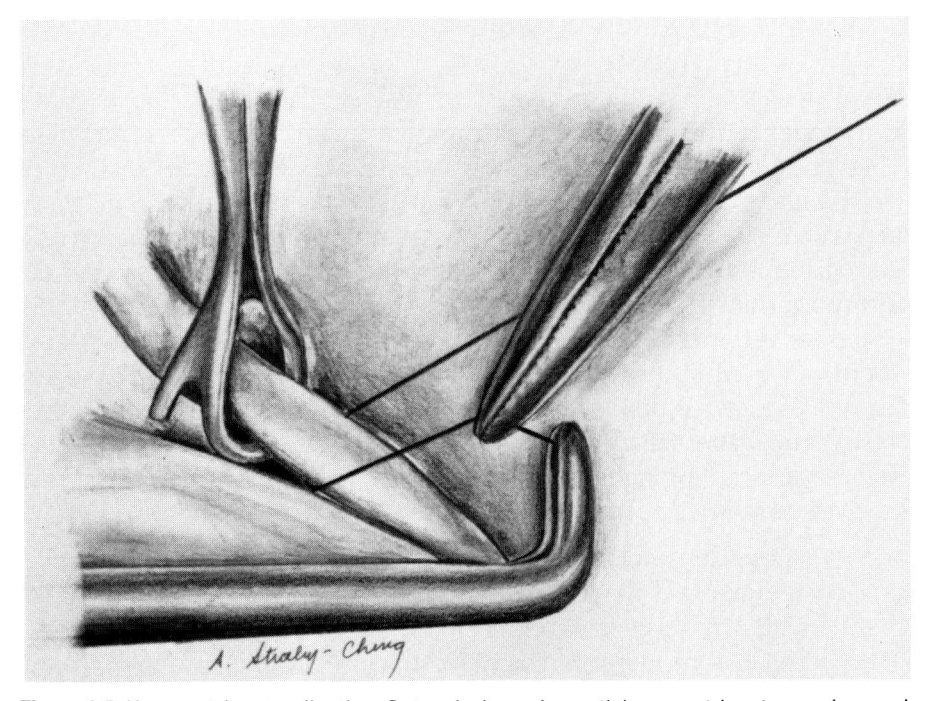

Figure 6.5 Hypogastric artery ligation. Suture is drawn beneath hypogastric artery and passed to tonsil clamp for second pass.

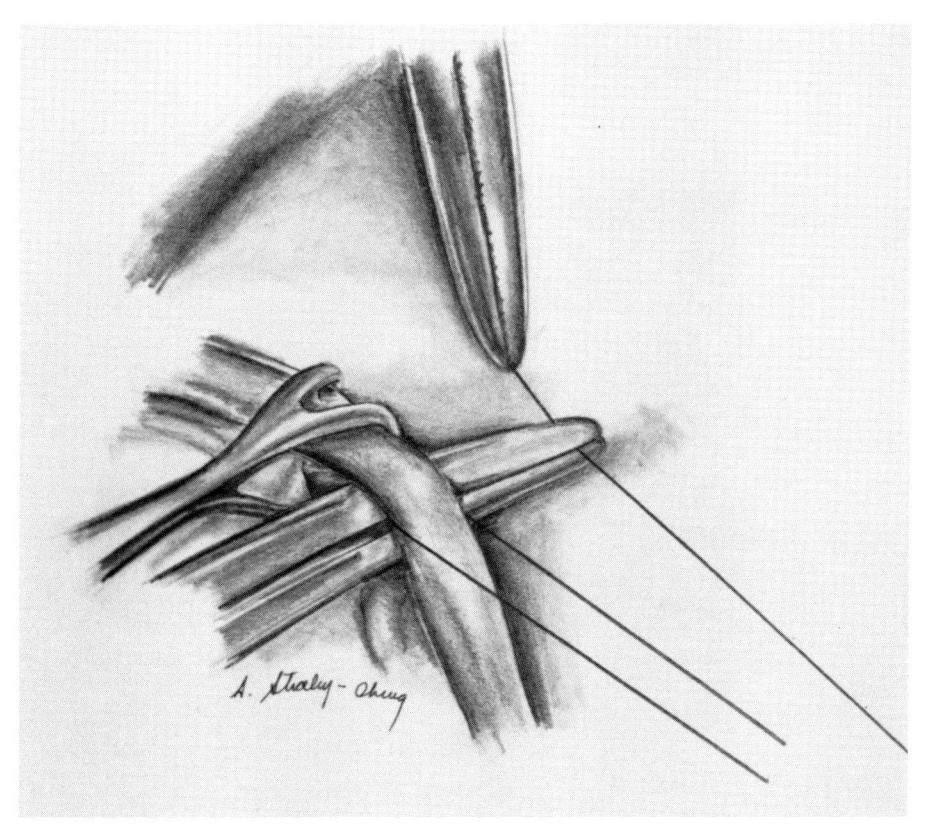

Figure 6.6 Hypogastric artery ligation. Mixter clamp is repositioned below hypogastric artery and suture on tonsil clamp is brought down and grasped by Mixter clamp for second pass below hypogastric artery.

hypogastric artery, however, is delay in its performance. This procedure does not overcome irreversible hemorrhagic shock.

It is generally agreed that this operation does not result in necrosis of vital pelvic structures or cutaneous areas and, other than surgical complications, there are no major complications following hypogastric artery ligation. The success rate of hypogastric artery ligation is difficult to assess. Approximately half of the patients with hemorrhage will respond successfully.[44] Suggestions as to why bilateral hypogastric artery ligation sometimes fails in controlling pelvic hemorrhage have included destruction of vessels from massive necrosis after infection, the presence of large aberrant branches that supply blood to the pelvic area, dislodging clots when blood pressure rises, and concomitant severe venous bleeding.

Angiographic Arterial Embolization

Angiographic arterial embolization[45–48] may be used as an alternative to bilateral hypogastric artery ligation in cases of uncontrollable pelvic hemorrhage. In effect the procedure produces a "nonsurgical" hypogastric

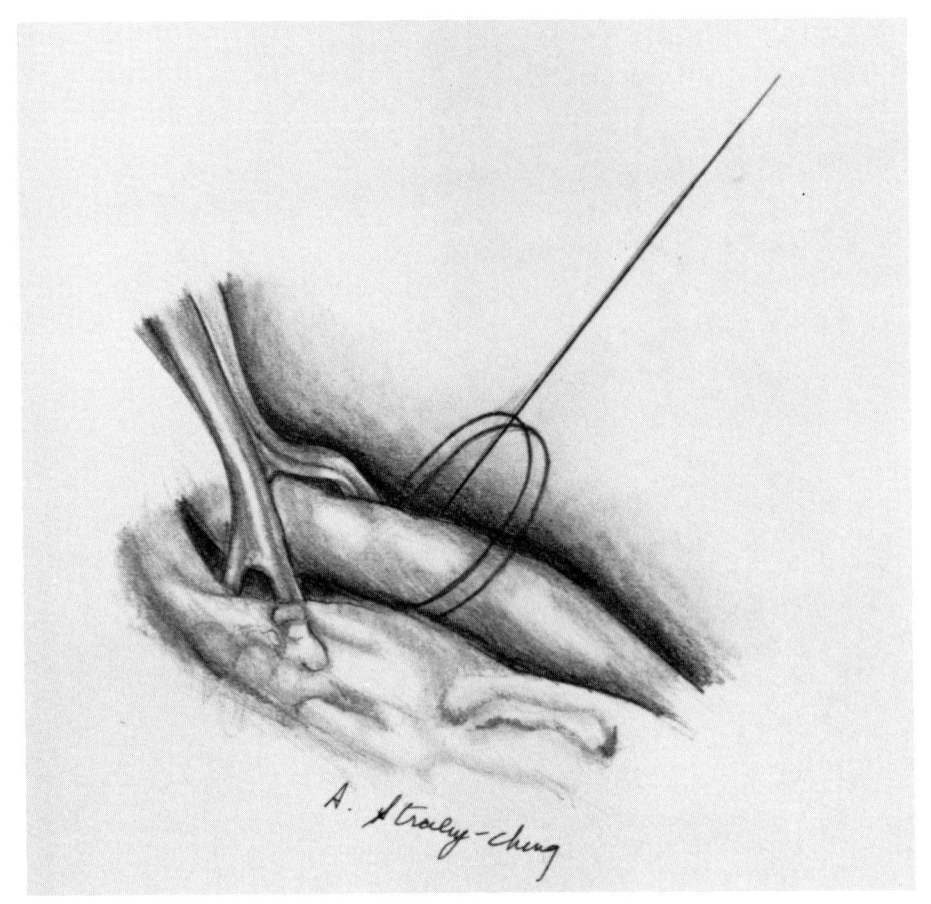

Figure 6.7 Hypogastric artery ligation. Double loop of suture is in position around hypogastric artery.

artery ligation. Its use for posthysterectomy bleeding not controlled by reoperative procedures is well documented.[48] Angiographers recommend that the surgeon request an angiographic consultation early. A patient who is reasonably stable and has not undergone reoperation is preferred because of the added technical simplicity and higher success rate. The key to successful embolization is accurate identification of the bleeding vessel. Previous hypogastric artery ligation makes embolization more difficult. Conversely, failure of embolization does not compromise the possibility of subsequent surgery. It should be remembered, however, that embolization requires 1 to 2 hours, so that, in severe hypotensive shock, it is not an appropriate option.

The procedure may be performed transfemorally, transbrachially, or directly into the aorta. The selection of transcatheter embolization agent is determined by the duration of desired occlusion, the size of the vessel to be occluded, the rate of blood flow through the vessel, and whether

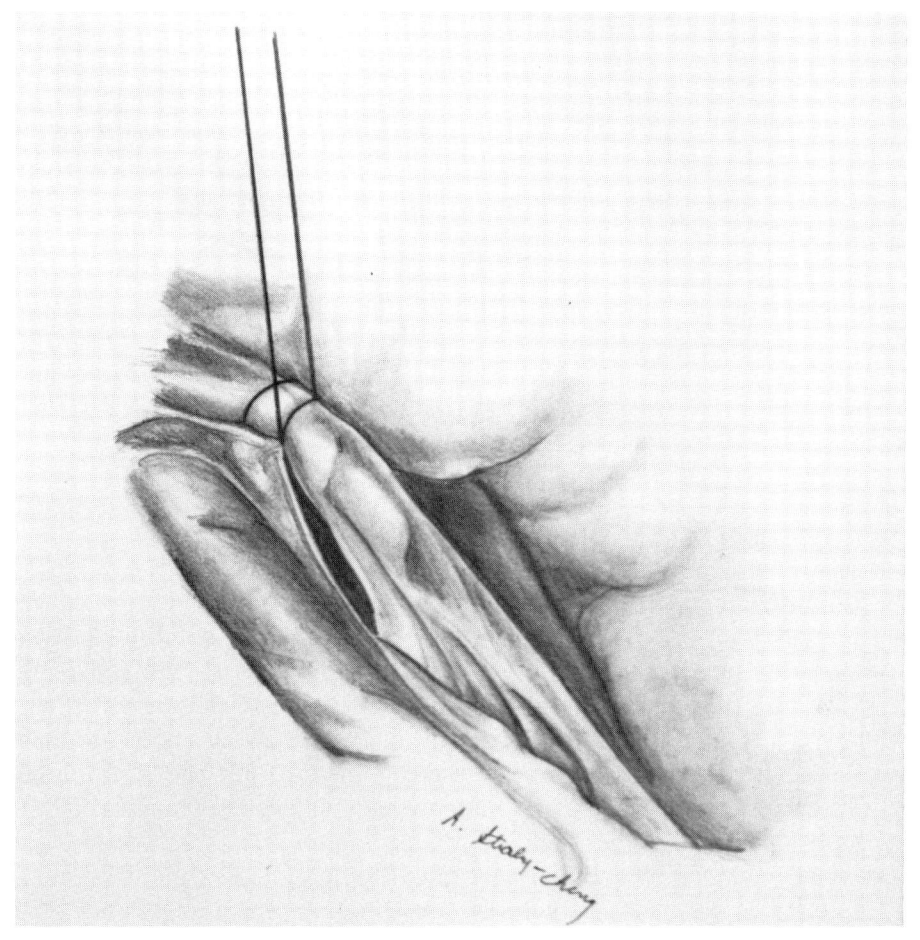

Figure 6.8 Hypogastric artery ligation. The doubly-passed suture has been moved to the bifurcation of the common iliac artery and is ready to be tied.

or not the vessel tapers or branches.[47] Absorbable gelatin sponge (Gelfoam), as small pledgets, is used to occlude small tapering vessels for short-term (10 to 30 days) occlusion. Larger, nontapering vessels are occluded with a detachable balloon or Gianturco coil.

Military Antishock Trousers

Military antishock trousers (MAST) can be a truly life-saving adjunct in the management of pelvic hemorrhage when other measures have failed. Hemorrhagic situations in which the MAST have been employed successfully include rupture of the liver in pregnancy, ruptured ectopic pregnancy, postcesarean hysterectomy, DIC, intractable intraoperative bleeding, and bleeding following radical pelvic surgery.[49]

Patients placed in the MAST respond with a decreased blood loss and rise in blood pressure as a consequence of increased peripheral resistance in the vessels. This effect allows for improved perfusion of critical organs such as the heart, lungs, brain, and kidneys, and may prevent irreversible shock, adult respiratory distress syndrome, and acute tubular necrosis. Patients with secondary coagulopathies in whom surgical intervention has failed to control bleeding are prime candidates for the use of MAST because this provides time to correct coagulation-related bleeding disorders.

Once the MAST are applied, they are inflated from the legs to the abdominal compartment with 10 to 40 mm Hg pressure to establish a stable perfusion and decrease bleeding. The MAST are removed 12 to 14 hours after the bleeding has ceased by deflating the abdominal compartment first, followed by the legs in 5-mm Hg increments every half hour.[50]

Posthysterectomy Bleeding

Postoperative hemorrhage may complicate any operative procedure regardless of how simple or extensive. Approximately 0.8% of hysterectomies[51] are complicated by postoperative hemorrhage requiring reoperation. Although it may be difficult to diagnose inapparent postoperative intraabdominal bleeding, any of the following should arouse suspicion: excessive postoperative pain; persistent oliguria; abdominal rigidity or distention; vaginal, shoulder, or scapular pain; tachycardia; or hypotension. Serial evaluations of the hemoglobin and hematocrit, ultrasound, culdocentesis, or an abdominal tap may aid in the diagnosis. If the index of suspicion is high, even without supporting evidence, celiotomy with complete exploration of the abdomen is always the next step.

Hysterectomy techniques that extraperitonealize vascular pedicles, leaving the vaginal cuff open, increase the likelihood that postoperative bleeding will be recognized earlier. Bleeding that is retroperitoneal or intraabdominal, without access to the vagina, is usually diagnosed after the patient has lost a significant volume of blood. In 1,219 vaginal hysterectomies reported by Smith and Pratt,[52] seven patients who required reoperation for hemorrhage developed symptoms 5 to 11 hours postoperatively. On physical examination, the patient will present with a distended abdomen with decreased bowel sounds or differential dullness on percussion that may or may not shift, the latter being true of retroperitoneal bleeding. Ultrasound scanning may be useful in locating the site of a hematoma but, ultimately, the discovery is made by reoperation.

Although the most common site of significant postoperative bleeding following hysterectomies is the vaginal vault, any vascular pedicle may be implicated. Patients evidencing postoperative bleeding within the first 24 hours generally bleed from a pedicle that was either inadequately sutured or in which suture breakage or slippage occurred. Bleeding after the first 24 hours is usually due to tissue or suture sloughing, but this etiology has decreased with the advent of synthetic absorbable sutures that retain their tensile strength up to 30 days.

Bleeding that occurs within the first 24 hours is best managed by appropriate reexploration and resuturing of the injured vessels. Those cases in which postoperative bleeding is more indolent (eg, presenting as a hematoma, both confined and self-tamponading) may require either reoperation or simply observation. Hematoma evacuation and placement of hemostatic sutures diminish the risk of secondary infection and abscess formation. However, many hematomas may self-tamponade and stabilize without additional bleeding or subsequent infection. The risk of infection relates to the indication for the original surgery, the use of antibiotics, and the general metabolic status of the patient.

Postoperative hemorrhage of significance is most often arterial in origin and must always be controlled surgically. The first step in its management is hemodynamic stabilization. An initial examination should be attempted before anesthesia and surgery, especially if bleeding per vagina is noted. With the patient in a lithotomy position, clots are removed and the vaginal cuff is examined. If a bleeding vessel is identified at or near the cuff, one or more superficial sutures may be adequate. If bleeding is extensive or originates above the vaginal apex, exploratory laparotomy becomes mandatory. Once the decision is made to explore the patient, a midline incision of sufficient size should be made to facilitate adequate exploration of all pelvic and abdominal structures. After evacuating all clots, exploration of the abdomen, along with careful examination of all previous pedicle sites, will usually suffice and allow for religature. The cyclic spurting of blood from arteries, as compared to a diffuse venous ooze that does not allow for clamping, facilitates their location and allows for precise clamping with a Tonsil clamp. Again, it should be emphasized that, regardless of the severity of bleeding, blind, haphazard clamping and suturing of tissues must be avoided. Direct compression with a finger or pack and slow release of the compression will aid in accurate clamp and suture placement. These conventional steps are lifesaving techniques that will resolve most cases. If the bleeding is diffuse or the bleeding vessels are located deep in the pelvis where they either cannot be located or, if located, are not amenable to suturing, the techniques of pelvic packing, hypogastric artery ligation, percutaneous embolization, or the use of MAST may be required.

Conclusion

Most gynecologists have had a routine procedure transformed into a life-threatening situation. The surgeon's attitude may be the deciding factor in the final outcome of these situations. Although fear is a normal reaction, the surgeon must keep a clear head even in the face of massive hemorrhage. Furthermore, the surgeon should recognize when the situation is drawing him or her away from the boundaries of knowledge and training. It is a wise individual who has a realistic appraisal of his or her abilities and seeks assistance when necessary. Finally, the goal of the pelvic surgeon should be prevention of hemorrhage by a complete and confident grasp of pelvic anatomy coupled with meticulous surgical technique.[53]

References

1. Best LC, Holland TK, Jones PB, et al: The interrelationship between thromboxane biosynthesis, aggregation and 5-hydroxytryptamine secretion in human platelets in vitro. *Thromb Haemost* 1980;43:38–40.
2. Addonizio VP Jr, Wetstein L, Fisher CA, et al: Mediation of cardiac ischemia by thromboxanes released from human platelets. *Surgery* 1982;92:292–298.
3. Schrier S: Disorders of hemostasis and coagulation, in Rubenstein E, Federman D (eds): *Scientific American Medicine.* New York, Scientific American Inc, 1988, pp 1–49.
4. Sharp AA: Diagnosis and management of disseminated intravascular coagulation. *Br Med Bull* 1977;33:265–272.
5. Addonizio VP, Stahl RF: Bleeding, in Wilmore DW, Brennan MR, Harken AL, et al (eds): *American College of Surgeons Care of the Surgical Patient.* New York, Scientific American Inc, 1989, pp 1–13.
6. Robboy SJ, Mihm MC, Colman BW, et al: The skin in disseminated intravascular coagulation: Prospective analysis of thirty-six cases. *Br J Dermatol* 1973;88:221–229.
7. McGehee WG, Rapaport SI, Hjort PF: Intravascular coagulation in fulminant meningococcemia. *Ann Intern Med* 1967;67:250–260.
8. Robboy SJ, Minna JD, Colman RW: Pulmonary hemorrhage syndrome as a manifestation of disseminated intravascular coagulation: Analysis of ten cases. *Chest* 1973;63:718–721.
9. Goldfinger D: Acute hemolytic transfusion reactions—a fresh look at pathogenesis and considerations regarding therapy. *Transfusion* 1977;17:85–98.
10. Counts RB, Haish C, Simon TL, et al: Hemostasis in massively transfused trauma patients. *Ann Surg* 1979;190:91–99.
11. Ingram GIC: The bleeding complications of blood transfusions. *Transfusion* 1965;5:1–5.
12. Bachmann F, Orranoot P: Surgical bleeding. *Med Clin North Am* 1972;56:207–219.
13. Bunker IF, Goldstein R: Coagulation during hypothermia in man. *Proc Soc Exp Biol Med* 1958;97:199–202.
14. Collins JA: Massive blood transfusion. *Clin Haematol* 1976;5:201–222.
15. Valeri CR, Cassity G, Khuri S, et al: Hypothermia-inducted reversible platelet dysfunction. *Ann Surg* 1987;205:175–181.
16. Antimicrobials and haemostasis [editorial]. *Lancet* 1983;1:510–511.
17. Weitekamp MR, Aber RC: Prolonged bleeding times and bleeding diathesis associated with moxalactam administration. *JAMA* 1983;249:69–71.

18. Lazarchick J, Hoyer LW: Immunoradiometric measurement of the factor VIII procoagulant antigen. *J Clin Invest* 1978;62:1048–1052.
19. Ingram GIC: Investigation of a long-standing bleeding tendency. *Br Med Bull* 1977;33:261–264.
20. Nilsson IM, Holmberg L: Von Willebrand's disease today. *Clin Haematol* 1979; 8:147.
21. Perry GS III, Spector BD, Schuman LM, et al: The Wiskott-Aldrich syndrome in the United States and Canada (1892–1979). *J Pediatr* 1980;97:72–78.
22. Weiss HJ: Platelet physiology and abnormalities of platelet function (pt 1). *N Engl J Med* 1975;293:531–541.
23. Clagett GP, Olsen WR: Nonmechanical hemorrhage in severe liver injury. *Ann Surg* 1978;187:369–374.
24. Counts RB, Haisch C, Simon TL, et al: Hemostasis in massively transfused trauma patients. *Ann Surg* 1979;190:91.
25. Kravans JR, Jackson DP: Hemorrhagic disorder following massive whole blood transfusion. *JAMA* 1955;159:171–177.
26. Lim RC, Olcott C, Robinson AJ, et al: Platelet response and coagulation changes following massive blood replacement. *J Trauma* 1973;13:577–582.
27. Miller RD, Robbins TO, Tong MJ, et al: Coagulation defects associated with massive blood transfusions. *Ann Surg* 1971;174:794–801.
28. Wilson RF, Mammen E, Walt AJ: Eight years of experience with massive blood transfusions. *J Trauma* 1971;11:275–285.
29. Lucas CE: Resuscitation of the injured patient: The three phases of treatment. *Surg Clin North Am* 1977;57:3–15.
30. Ciavarella D, Reed RL, Counts RB, et al: Clotting factor levels and the risk of diffuse microvascular bleeding. *Br J Haematol* 1987;67:365–368.
31. Mannucci PM, Federici AB, Sirchi DG: Hemostasis testing during massive blood replacement: A study of 172 cases. *Vox Sang* 1982;42:113–123.
32. Nolan TE, Gallup DG: Massive transfusion: A current review. *Obstet Gynecol Surv* 1991;46:289–295.
33. Consensus conference: Fresh-frozen plasma: Indications and risks. *JAMA* 1985;253:551–553.
34. Barik SS, Dogra M, Khunnu B, et al: Inferior vena cava ligation for intractable pelvic hemorrhage. *Aust N Z J Obstet Gynaecol* 1990;30:86–87.
35. Breen JL, Kindzierski J, Gregori C: *Hemorrhage in Gynecologic Surgery* (Current Therapy in Surgical Gynecology). Philadelphia, BC Decker, 1987.
36. Logothetopulos K: Eine absolut sichere Blutstillungs methode bei vaginalen und abdominalen gynakologischen operationen. *Zentralbl Gynaekol* 1926; 50:3202–3204.
37. Guerre EF, O'Keefe DF, Elliot JP, et al: Uncontrollable intra-abdominal hemorrhage treated with packing and use of a MAST suit. *J Reprod Med* 1987; 32:230–232.
38. Reich WJ, Nichtow MJ: Ligation of the internal iliac (hypogastric) arteries: A lifesaving procedure for uncontrollable gynecologic and obstetric hemorrhage. *J Int Coll Surg* 1961;36:157–168.
39. Sagarra M, Glasser T, Stone ML: Ligation of the internal iliac vessels in the control of post partum hemorrhage. *Obstet Gynecol* 1960;15:698–701.
40. Breen JI, DeLia J: Control of surgical hemorrhage, in Nichols D (ed): *Reoperative Gynecologic Surgery*. St. Louis, Mosby-Year Book, 1991.

41. Goss CM (ed): *Gray's Anatomy,* ed 29. Philadelphia, Lea & Febiger, 1973.
42. Burchell RC: Internal iliac artery ligation: Aortograms. *Obstet Gynecol* 1966; 94:117–124.
43. Burchell RC: Internal iliac artery ligation: Hemodynamics. *Obstet Gynecol* 1964;24:737–739.
44. Clark SL, Phelan JP, Yen S, et al: Hypogastric artery ligation for obstetrical hemorrhage. *Acta Obstet Gynecol Scand* 1985;66:353–356.
45. Brown BJ, Heaston DK, Poulson AM, et al: Uncontrollable postpartum bleeding: A new approach to hemostasis through angiographic arterial embolization. *Obstet Gynecol* 1979;54:361–365.
46. Kivikoski AI, Matin C, Weyman PJ, et al: Angiographic arterial embolization to control hemorrhage in abdominal pregnancy: A case report. *Obstet Gynecol* 1988;71:456–459.
47. Marx MV, Picus D, Weyman PJ: Percutaneous embolization of the ovarian artery in the treatment of pelvic hemorrhage. *Am J Radiol* 1988;150:1337–1338.
48. Rosenthal DM, Colapinto R: Angiographic arterial embolization in the management of postoperative vaginal hemorrhage. *Am J Obstet Gynecol* 1985; 151:227–231.
49. Hall M, Marshall JR: The gravity suit: A major advance in management of gynecologic blood loss. *Obstet Gynecol* 1979;53:247–250.
50. Kaback KR, Sanders AB, Meislin HW: MAST suit update. *JAMA* 1984;252:2598–2603.
51. Fegrman H: Surgical management of life threatening obstetric and gynecologic hemorrhage. *Acta Obstet Gynecol Scand* 1988;67:125–128.
52. Smith RD, Pratt JH: Serious bleeding following vaginal or abdominal hysterectomy. *Obstet Gynecol* 1965;26:592–595.
53. Breen JL, Gregori C, Denehy T: Hemorrhage, ACOG Obstetrics and Gynecology Audio-visual Tape #1. Anaheim, CA, American College of Obstetrics and Gynecology, 1991.

Chapter 7

Controversial Techniques During Hysterectomy

Thomas G. Stovall, MD

Much has been written and taught about vaginal hysterectomy and specific techniques used during the procedure. Too often, we as gynecologic surgeons accept what is written at face value without examining the objective data behind such statements. Thus, the purpose of this chapter is to review some of the specific techniques used by gynecologic surgeons during hysterectomy and examine the data that exist or do not exist to support the use of these techniques.

Uterine Morcellation During Vaginal Hysterectomy

The preoperative indication for the majority of hysterectomies performed in the United States is leiomyomata uteri, with most of these hysterectomies being approached abdominally.[1] If there is to be a significant increase in the number of patients in whom the vaginal approach is used, a change in our surgical thinking when dealing with the symptomatic large uterus is mandatory. Vaginal hysterectomy by morcellation is a well-known, but often underutilized surgical procedure. Several methods for uterine morcellation, or piecemeal uterine removal, have been described. These include hemisection or bivalving, wedge/"V"-type incisions, and intramyometrial coring/Lash procedure.[2]

Hemisection/Bivalving

Hemisection of the uterus has been described but is an infrequently used method of morcellation.[3] Utilizing this technique, the cervix is split in the midline and the uterine fundus is cut into halves. One side of the uterine specimen is removed, and then the other. This method seems best suited for the fundal, midline fibroid. This technique is probably used less frequently than the other methods described.

Wedge Morcellation

"Wedge" morcellation is begun by amputating the cervix and grasping the myometrium with a Leahy clamp or tenaculum. Wedge-shaped morcels of myometrium are removed from the anterior and/or posterior uterine wall. The apex of the wedge is directed to the midline, thereby reducing the bulk of the myometrium. The excision is continued until the uterus can be removed, or until a pseudocapsule of a fibroid is reached. The fibroid can be grasped with a Leahy clamp or towel clip, traction applied, and a myomectomy performed. This technique is best suited for anterior or posterior fibroids or for fibroids in one or the other broad ligament away from the midline.

Lash Procedure/Intramyometrial Coring

The uterus is converted from a globular to an elongated tissue mass.[4,5] The "cored" uterus is then removed by clamping the uteroovarian pedicles and fallopian tubes. Once the uterosacral and cardinal ligaments and uterine vessels have been ligated and the pedicles secured, the myometrium, above the ligated vessels, is incised circumferentially parallel to the axis of the uterine cavity and serosa. The surgeon must utilize caution not to extend the scalpel through the uterine serosa. The incision is continued around the full circumference of the myometrium in a symmetric fashion beneath the serosa of the uterus. Traction should be maintained on the cervix to facilitate the procedure and to reduce blood loss. The myometrium is cut so that the endometrial cavity is not entered. Incising the lateral portions of the myometrium medial to the remaining attachment of the broad ligament results in uterine descent and mobility.

Combination of Methods

Not every operative encounter is suited for a single type of uterine morcellation procedure. More commonly, one or more of the above methods in combination are used. Table 7.1 provides specific techniques that we have found helpful when uterine morcellation is contemplated.

Feasibility/Safety of Uterine Morcellation Combined with Vaginal Hysterectomy

Two large studies have reported the author's extensive experience with uterine morcellation at the time of vaginal hysterectomy. Kovac, in 1986,[6] compared three groups of patients in an attempt to determine the safety of uterine morcellation. Group I ($n = 554$) was composed of patients undergoing vaginal hysterectomy with intramyometrial coring, with (38.6%) or without (61.4%) anterior or posterior colporrhaphy. Group II ($n = 173$) was composed of patients undergoing vaginal hysterectomy

Table 7.1 Procedural Tips for Uterine Morcellation

1. Patient positioning and lighting are very important.
2. Interested assistants are mandatory.
3. Retractors to be used include: malleable ribbon, Deaver retractor and Steiner-Anvard posterior-weighted speculum with elongated tip.
4. Heaney needle holder use is recommended
5. Patients should also give consent for abdominal hysterectomy.
6. Prophylactic antibiotics in a single preoperative dose are used.
7. No excess vaginal mucosa is removed.
8. Traction should be maintained throughout the procedure to decrease blood loss.
9. The peritoneal cavity should be entered before beginning morcellation.
10. Uterosacral cardinal ligaments and uterine arteries should be clamped prior to beginning morcellation.
11. A Beaver knife facilitates myometrial cutting.

without coring, and group III ($n = 175$) consisted of patients undergoing abdominal hysterectomy.

Patients in groups I and III were more likely to be operated on for leiomyomata, and patients with a preoperative indication of pelvic inflammatory disease were more likely to be operated on abdominally (group III). The mean uterine weight in the uterine morcellation group was 163 (range 100 to 750) g. The mean operative time of 40 (range 15 to 110) minutes in Group I compared favorably to the 68 (range 30 to 280) minutes in the abdominal hysterectomy group. Febrile morbidity was not significantly different in any of the three groups. The transfusion rate in group I of 2.9% was higher than in those patients undergoing only vaginal hysterectomy (group II, 1.2%), but less than in those requiring abdominal hysterectomy (group III, 4.6%). Kovac concluded that vaginal hysterectomy was the technique of choice for the management of patients with nonmalignant pelvic disease and that uterine morcellation was a safe procedure.

Grody[7] reviewed 324 consecutive cases of vaginal hysterectomy for uteri weighing 190 to 810 g in which uterine morcellation was used. In this series, bladder injury occurred in only four patients (0% to 12%). The mean hospital stay was 3.8 (range 2 to 6) days and decreased to 3.3 days during the last 15 years of the study. Febrile morbidity occurred in 16% of patients but decreased to 10% when preoperative antibiotics and synthetic sutures were used, and hemorrhage requiring transfusion occurred in 14%. Grody concluded that, when hysterectomy is indicated, the vaginal route should be considered first and, when feasible, the surgery should be performed by gynecologic surgeons who are capable of doing this procedure. Both of these studies report the experience of a single operating surgeon with a great deal of experience in vaginal surgery. Although these studies point to the feasibility of vaginal removal of the large uterus, neither study had reproducible criteria for selecting candidates for vaginal hysterectomy, and neither was a prospective randomized trial. However, even with these limitations, it appears that uterine morcellation and vaginal removal of the large uterus are safe and have a place in gynecologic surgery.

Luteinizing Hormone–Releasing Hormone Agonists and Hysterectomy

Myomas are highly responsive to estrogen stimulation, a fact supported by their rapid growth during pregnancy and their tendency to become smaller following menopause. Since leiomyomata appear to be estrogen-dependent to varying degrees, suppressing intrinsic estrogen production should logically result in size reduction. Luteinizing hormone–releasing hormone (LH-RH) agonists have the ability to induce a hypoestrogen state without causing intrinsic steroidal effects, and are therefore an excellent drug to reduce myoma size during the preoperative period. Table 7.2 provides a summary of the results when LH-RH agonists are given to a patient with leiomyomata.[8-11]

A review of the literature and other chapters in this book clearly establish: (1) the benefits of vaginal hysterectomy over abdominal hysterectomy, (2) the safety and efficacy of uterine morcellation, and (3) the reduction of myoma size by LH-RH agonists. However, many practicing gynecologic surgeons do not recommend vaginal hysterectomy when the uterus is larger than the equivalent of 10 to 14 weeks' gestation. In view of these issues, one must consider whether a short course of preoperative LH-RH agonist prior to planned hysterectomy for leiomyomata uteri could result in an increased utilization of vaginal hysterectomy, and whether such treatment would be associated with a decrease in morbidity, hospital stay, or convalescent period. Such a study was performed at the University of Tennessee in Memphis.[12]

Fifty premenopausal patients requiring hysterectomy for symptomatic, 14- to 18-week gestation equivalent size leiomyomata uteri were

Table 7.2 Summary of the Effects of LH-RH Agonists on Leiomyomata Uteri

1. Successful size reduction in 95% of myomata, with an expected reduction in volume of 50–60%.
2. Maximum reduction in size occurs during the first 12 wk of treatment, with the maximum slope of reduction occurring between 4 and 8 wk of treatment.
3. An increase in size occurs after treatment in 95% of cases.
4. Hot flashes diminish in frequency and intensity after several weeks of treatment, but are the most common complaints of patients.
5. Bone and lipid effects with short-course therapy are negligible and, if they were to occur, are reversible.
6. Amenorrhea is induced in over 95% of patients, with a resulting increase in hemoglobin and hematocrit.
7. Approximately 1% of patients experience myoma degeneration with profuse vaginal bleeding, necessitating prompt surgical intervention.

Table 7.3 Data Summary for Patients Randomized to Hysterectomy With or Without Preoperative LH-RH Agonist

Characteristics Studied	Group A: Control Group ($n = 25$)	Group B: Preoperative LH-RH Agonist ($n = 25$)	p Value[a]
Mean preoperative hemoglobin (g/dL)	11.17 ± 2.0 (8.1–15.2)	10.75 ± 2.2 (6.7–14.3)	NS
Mean pretreatment uterine size (wk gestation equivalent)	15.4 ± 1.2 (14–18)	15.7 ± 1.4 (14–18)	NS
Mean preoperative exam, uterine size (wk gestation equivalent)	15.4 ± 1.2 (14–18)	11.4 ± 1.6 (9–14)	.0001
Pretreatment ultrasonographic uterine volume (mL)	888.4 ± 520.1 (356–2145)	1086.7 ± 582.4 (414–2138)	NS
Mean preoperative ultrasonic uterine volume (mL)	888.4 ± 520.1 (360–2145)	723.4 ± 296.9 (280–1305)	NS
Procedure performed			
Abdominal hysterectomy	21 (84%)	6 (24%)	<.05
Vaginal hysterectomy	4 (16%)	18 (76%)	<.05
Mean operative time, (min)	104.2 ± 29.5 (57–163)	93.1 ± 41.9 (40–145)	NS
Mean operative blood loss (mL)	613.9 ± 108.0 (131–1583)	527 ± 73.9 (110–1020)	.042[a]
Mean postoperative hospital stay (d)	5.2 ± 1.8 (4–11)	3.8 ± 1.9 (2–10)	.022[a]

[a] $p < .05$ concluded as significant.

randomized into two groups to determine if preoperative LH-RH agonist would increase the feasibility of vaginal rather than abdominal hysterectomy. The control group (group A; $n = 25$) did not receive preoperative LH-RH agonist, whereas patients in group B ($n = 25$) received 2 months of LH-RH agonist prior to hysterectomy (Table 7.3). Patients in the two groups were similar with respect to age, gravidity, parity, pretreatment uterine size, and hemoglobin/hematocrit levels. Patients in group B demonstrated an increase in hemoglobin levels (10.75 to 12.12 g/dL; $p < .05$) and a decrease in uterine volume (1086.7 to 723.4 mL; $p < .05$) after 8 weeks of agonist therapy, and were more likely to undergo vaginal hysterectomy (76% versus 16%). When compared with group A, patients in group B also had shorter hospitalization (5.2 versus 3.8 days; $p < .05$).

The cost of 2 months of leuprolide acetate therapy at our institution ranges from $350.00 to $600.00 depending on whether patients are able to share the cost of a vial of drug, and/or whether the patient chooses to use the daily injection or the depot formulation. This cost, however, is offset by a decreased length of hospital stay and a decreased length of convalescence, thus reducing time lost from work. In the future, additional studies may show that estrogen replacement therapy can also be utilized in combination with LH-RH agonist therapy to decrease the hypoestrogenic side effects associated with this therapy without offsetting the benefits of uterine size reduction.

This study demonstrated that selected premenopausal patients with leiomyomata uteri of 14 to 18 weeks' gestation equivalent size can safely undergo vaginal hysterectomy when treated with a short course of LH-RH agonists prior to surgery. This method seems preferable to abdominal hysterectomy, which these patients otherwise would have undergone, because it is associated with a shorter postoperative hospital stay and an overall decrease in the convalescent period following surgery. Based on the results of this study, it appears that preoperative LH-RH agonist therapy for 2 months prior to planned vaginal hysterectomy for the patient with leiomyomata uteri of 14 to 18 weeks' gestation equivalent size, and for the patient with a preoperative hematocrit of less than 30%, is acceptable.

Outpatient Vaginal Hysterectomy

Over the last 10 years, there has been a vast expansion in the types and numbers of patients on whom operations are performed on an outpatient basis. As an extension of this pattern, a study was conducted to determine the feasibility and safety of vaginal hysterectomy when performed as an outpatient procedure. Stovall et al[13] conducted a prospective study of 35 patients between January and July, 1991. Inclusion criteria required that the patient: (1) have no medical problems requiring hospitalization, (2) have a working telephone and a support person during the first 48 postoperative hours, (3) sign an informed consent and have an understanding of the postoperative instructions, (4) not require a concomitant surgical procedure such as anterior or posterior colporrhaphy, (5) not require additional antibiotic prophylaxis, and (6) not sustain an intraoperative injury requiring hospital monitoring. Following hospital discharge, all patients were seen in their home on postoperative days 1 and 2 by a visiting nurse, who obtained vital signs, complete blood count, and serum electrolytes. In addition, a physician contacted the patient by phone on the evening of surgery and on postoperative days 1 and 2 to review the patient's temperature record and pain control. Patients were seen at 1 and 6 weeks in the outpatient clinic. Total hospital stay from admission to discharge from the ambulatory surgery unit was 9.4 ± 0.81 (range 7.8 to 10.6) hours. The mean preoperative hematocrit was $37.0\% \pm 3.5$ (range 29.3 to 43.5), with a mean discharge hematocrit of $32.5\% \pm 4.2$ (range 27 to 39.0). An oxycodone/acetaminophen combination was used for pain control during the first postoperative week. Hematocrits done at 24 hours, 48 hours, and 1 week were unchanged ($p < .05$) from the hematocrit obtained at the time of hospital discharge. Two patients required hospital readmission; the first was readmitted on postoperative day 7 for a vaginal cuff abscess and the second on postoperative day 3 for a spinal headache. Results of a 13-item questionnaire indicated that the majority of patients rated the entire outpatient experience positively.

Subsequently, the experience has been expanded to now include over 100 patients who have been discharged on the day of surgery following vaginal hysterectomy. These data suggest that outpatient vaginal hysterectomy can be a safe procedure, and is well accepted by selected patients. Additional studies will be required to determine if this can become a feasible alternative for a greater number of patients.

Issues Related to Enterocele and Vault Prolapse Prevention

Vaginal vault prolapse can follow either transvaginal or transabdominal hysterectomy, with an occurrence of approximately 1%. Prevention, if possible, is generally not emphasized. However, several methods have been described, including the McCall[14] culdoplasty and the attachment of the cardinal ligaments and/or the uterosacral ligaments to the vagina.[15] Suture approximation of the round ligaments to the vagina wall has also been proposed, but this may lead to dyspareunia as a result of the ovaries being brought into closer approximation to the vaginal cuff. In a report dealing with posthysterectomy enterocele and vaginal vault prolapse, Symmonds et al[16] stated that, of 60 patients with vault prolapse after vaginal hysterectomy, 39 were operated on using the Mayo or Mayo-Ward operative technique, which does not include uterosacral plication. However, since, 1956 at the Mayo Clinic, all patients undergoing vaginal hysterectomy were operated on using a modified Heaney technique combined with a prophylactic culdoplasty. It was Symmonds et al's clinical impression at the time that the incidence of vault prolapse and enterocele formation had been greatly reduced. Although this clinical impression may indeed be correct, it has not been reported as such and has not been substantiated in a prospective randomized trial in which a comparison group of women was followed longitudinally. It is only through improved reporting of well-developed studies that truly appropriate and necessary surgical technique can be shown to be beneficial.

Vaginal Cuff Closure at Vaginal Hysterectomy

Numerous methods of vaginal cuff closure during vaginal hysterectomy have been described.[17] Major considerations include hemostasis and maintaining vaginal depth. Despite various recommendations made in various authoritative surgical texts, little has been published in this regard. Cruikshank[18] compared five methods of vaginal cuff closure in a prospective, randomized fashion in 112 patients undergoing vaginal hysterectomy. Patients were equally randomized to one of five methods of cuff closure: (1) horizontal, closed interrupted method; (2) horizontal closure with interrupted sutures laterally, while leaving the midportion open; (3) longitudinal closure using interrupted sutures to close the upper three fourths of the cuff, with the lower one fourth sutured with a continuous interlocking suture, leaving the cuff open; (4) longitudinal interrupted closure; and (5) longitudinal closure with a continuous interlocking suture. Cruikshank found no difference in morbidity or vaginal depth regardless of which method was used for vaginal mucosal reapproximation.

Peritoneal Closure at Vaginal Hysterectomy

Most gynecologic surgeons no longer close visceral or peritoneal peritoneum at the time of abdominal hysterectomy or cesarean section.[19,20] However, gynecologic textbooks and surgical atlases routinely describe closure of the peritoneum at the time of vaginal hysterectomy.[21-23] Ling et al[24] recently presented the results of a prospective trial in which patients were randomized to peritoneal closure ($N = 32$) or no peritoneal closure ($N = 28$) at the time of vaginal hysterectomy. The groups were similar with respect to age, gravidity, parity, and preoperative indication. The incidence of postoperative complication was also similar. Transvaginal ultrasound was used to measure the distance between the vaginal cuff and ovaries. In the patients who had peritoneal closure, the average distances of the right and left ovaries from the vaginal cuff were 1.57 ± 0.53 and 1.79 ± 0.61 cm, respectively. In the no-closure group, the right and left ovarian distances were 1.89 ± 0.69 and 1.66 ± 0.72 cm, respectively. Also, the incidence of deep-thrust dyspareunia was also similar in both groups. This study calls into question the necessity for reperitonealization at the time of vaginal hysterectomy.

Vasoconstrictivity Agent Use

In a time when great fear surrounds the need for transfusion of blood and blood products, the gynecologic surgeon is even more motivated in his or her attempt to keep blood loss to a minimum. In 1957, Lazar et al[25] reported the use of multiple-site infiltration in 190 vaginal hysterectomies using epinephrine. This study showed a significant reduction in blood loss during and after surgery when infiltration was used. In an additional report, Lazar[26] used the weight method to accurately determine the blood loss during vaginal surgery with and without the use of 1:1,000 epinephrine. A variety of surgical procedures was reported, including vaginal hysterectomy ($n = 80$) with and without anterior and posterior colporrhaphy, Manchester operations ($n = 20$), anterior and posterior colporrhaphy alone ($n = 57$), and Le Fort operations ($n = 5$). In the group of patients undergoing vaginal hysterectomy with and without colporrhaphy, the mean blood loss in the infiltration group was 305 mL, with 75% losing less than 400 mL. The average blood loss in the noninfiltrated group was 755 mL, with 90% losing over 400 mL. Additionally, no postoperative hemorrhage was reported in patients in whom infiltration was used. Lazar concluded that epinephrine infiltration was a safe procedure and one that should be used.

England et al[27] randomized 200 patients into two groups, with 100 patients receiving normal saline as a placebo control and 100 patients receiving epinephrine 1:200,000 injections circumferentially at the cervicovaginal junction before vaginal hysterectomy. A postoperative infection developed in 11% of the epinephrine-treated group and only 2% of the control group. Thus, the relative risk of developing a postoperative infection was 5.5 among patients in whom epinephrine was used. No statistical difference was noted in the number of patients requiring transfusions. Also, the mean change in venous hematocrit was -5.1% for the placebo group and -4.5% for the group in whom epinephrine was used. Thus, England et al concluded that the use of a vasoconstrictive agent at the time of vaginal hysterectomy could not be recommended. To date, this prospective, randomized trial presents the best data that we have at the present time and is the basis of why these authors do not use vasoconstrictive agents during vaginal hysterectomy.

Salpingo-Oophorectomy at Vaginal Hysterectomy

With the advent of the laparoscopic-assisted approach to vaginal hysterectomy, the role of transvaginal salpingo-oophorectomy must be viewed in a new light. Published information on the frequency with which adnexal removal can be accomplished with vaginal hysterectomy includes that of Smale et al,[28] who reported 485 vaginal hysterectomies, 355 of which included successful adnexal removal. Only one instance of postoperative hemorrhage from ovarian vessels was related to adnexal removal. In this series, no attempt was made to determine how many cases of adnexal removal were attempted but not completed. It does, however, demonstrate the safety and feasibility of adnexal removal at vaginal hysterectomy. Sheth[29] reported a series of 1,440 women undergoing vaginal hysterectomy, 740 of whom had attempted oophorectomy. Oophorectomy was possible in 702 (95%) of these patients; removal of one or both ovaries was not technically feasible in 38 patients (5%). Postoperative hospital stay and incidence of hemorrhage were similar in both groups. Obese patients, those who were nulliparous, and those with a subjective decrease in uterine descent or vaginal access, as well as those with tuboovarian disease, were less likely to have successful ovarian removal.

In another study, Hoffman[30] reported that only 4/20 (20%) patients had successful oophorectomies with the clamp technique. In 10/20 patients, bilateral oophorectomy could not be done with the clamp technique but was accomplished with the Endoloop technique, and in one patient one ovary was removed with the clamp technique and the other removed with Endoloops. One patient had only one of two ovaries successfully removed with an Endoloop, with the other ovary not being accessible. In the remaining four patients, safe transvaginal removal of the ovaries was not thought to be possible and was not attempted. These data do not support the necessity of abdominal hysterectomy for ovarian removal. It is sound gynecologic thinking to proceed with abdominal ovarian removal in the presence of adnexal disease. However, when prophylactic ovarian removal is warranted, the vaginal route is not contraindicated. These data also refute the idea of laparoscopic assistance being required at the time of hysterectomy. A more prudent approach might be attempted clamp or looped-suture removal while reserving laparoscopic removal only for those cases in which this cannot be accomplished. One must also factor in the small frequency with which ovarian pathology will occur if the ovaries are left in situ. This area of gynecologic surgical technique requires additional research.

Summary

When procedures or techniques used during vaginal hysterectomy are critically analyzed, it is readily apparent that much of what has been previously written or taught may have in fact been based on observation rather than clinical trials. Not every technique is applicable in all situations, nor should vaginal hysterectomy always be used to replace abdominal hysterectomy. However, when vaginal hysterectomy is used, the data reported here should be considered to determine the specific technical aspects of the operation.

References

1. Dicker RC, Greenspan JR, Strauss LT, et al: Complications of abdominal and vaginal hysterectomy among women of reproductive age in the United States: The Collaborative Review of Sterilization. *Am J Obstet Gynecol* 1982;144:841–847.
2. Pratt JH, Gunn H, Laugsson G: Vaginal hysterectomy by morcellation. *Mayo Clin Proc* 1970;45:374–387.
3. Nichols DH, Randall CL: *Vaginal Surgery*, ed 3. Baltimore, Williams and Wilkins, 1989, pp 204–214.
4. Lash AF: A method for reducing the size of the uterus in vaginal hysterectomy. *Am J Obstet Gynecol* 1941;42:452–458.
5. Lash AF: Technique for removal of abnormally large uteri without entering the cavities. *Clin Obstet Gynecol* 1961;4:210–215.

6. Kovac SR: Intramyometrial coring as an adjunct to vaginal hysterectomy. *Obstet Gynecol* 1986;67:131–136.
7. Grody MHT: Vaginal hysterectomy: The large uterus. *J Gynecol Surg* 1989;5:301–312.
8. Friedman AJ, Barbieri RL, Benecerraf BR, et al: Treatment of leiomyomata with intranasal or subcutaneous leuprolide, a gonadotropin-releasing hormone agonist. *Fertil Steril* 1987;48:560–564.
9. West CP, Lumsden MA, Lawson S, et al: Shrinkage of uterine fibroids during therapy with goserelin (Zoladex): A luteinizing hormone-releasing hormone agonist administered as a monthly subcutaneous depot. *Fertil Steril* 1987;48:45–51.
10. Coddington CC, Coddington RL, Shawker TH, et al: Long-acting gonadotropin hormone-releasing hormone analog used to treat uteri. *Fertil Steril* 1986;45:624–629.
11. Candiani GB, Vencellini P, Fedele L, et al: Use of goserelin depot, a gonadotropin-releasing hormone agonist, for the treatment of menorrhagia and severe anemia in women with leiomyomata uteri. *Acta Obstet Gynecol Scand* 1990;69:413–415.
12. Stovall TG, Ling FW, Henry LC, et al: A randomized trial evaluating leuprolide acetate prior to hysterectomy for leiomyomata. *Am J Obstet Gynecol* 1991;164:1420–1425.
13. Stovall TG, Summitt RL Jr, Bran DF, et al: Outpatient vaginal hysterectomy: A pilot study. *Obstet Gynecol*, 1992;80:143–150.
14. McCall ML: Posterior culdoplasty. *Obstet Gynecol* 1957;10:595–596.
15. Cruikshank SH: Preventing vault prolapse and enterocele after vaginal hysterectomy. *South Med J* 1988;81:594.
16. Symmonds RE, Williams TJ, Lee RA, et al: Posthysterectomy enterocele and vaginal vault prolapse. *Am J Obstet Gynecol* 1981;140:52–59.
17. Grossman RA: A new cuff closure technique for vaginal hysterectomy. *Am J Gynecol Health* 1988;2:30–32.
18. Cruikshank SH: Methods of vaginal cuff closure during vaginal hysterectomy. *South Med J* 1988;81:1375–1378.
19. Tulandi T, Hum HS, Gelfand MM: Closure of laparotomy incision with or without peritoneal suturing and second-look laparoscopy. *Am J Obstet Gynecol* 1988;158:536–537.
20. Hull DB, Varner MW: A randomized study of closure of the peritoneum at cesarean delivery. *Obstet Gynecol* 1991;77:818–820.
21. Smith HA, Thompson JD: Indications and techniques for vaginal hysterectomy, in Sanz LE (ed): *Gynecologic Surgery*, Cradell, NJ, Medical Economics Books, 1988, pp 140–151.
22. Thompson JD: Hysterectomy, in Thompson JD, Rock JA (eds): *TeLinde's Operative Gynecology*, ed 7. Phildelphia, JB Lippincott, 1992, pp 720–724.
23. Reiffenstuhl G, Platzer W: *Atlas of Vaginal Surgery: Surgical Anatomy and Technique*, Friedman JE, Friedman EA (trans), Friedman ED (ed). Phildelphia, WB Saunders, 1975, pp 214–280.
24. Ling FW, Stovall TG, Summitt RL Jr, et al: Peritoneal closure at the time of vaginal hysterectomy: A reassessment. Read at the meeting of the Society of Gynecologic Surgeons, March 3, 1992, Orlando, FL.
25. Lazar MR, Krieger HA: Blood loss in vaginal surgery: A comparative study. *Obstet Gynecol* 1959;13:707.

26. Lazar MR: Blood loss prevention in vaginal surgery. 1671–1677.
27. England GT, Randall HW, Graves WL: Impairment of tissue defenses by vasoconstrictors in vaginal hysterectomies. *Obstet Gynecol* 1983;61:271–274.
28. Smale LE, Smale ML, Wikening RL, et al: Salpingo-oophorectomy at the time of vaginal hysterectomy. *Am J Obstet Gynecol* 1978;131:122–128.
29. Sheth SS: The place of oophorectomy at vaginal hysterectomy. *Br J Obstet Gynaecol* 1991;98:662–666.
30. Hoffman MS: Transvaginal removal of ovaries with Endoloop suture at the time of transvaginal hysterectomy. *Am J Obstet Gynecol* 1991;165:407–408.

Chapter **8**

Additional Surgical Procedures at the Time of Hysterectomy

Robert L. Summitt, Jr, MD

Hysterectomy is one of the few operations in medicine with which concomitant surgical procedures are frequently performed. In many cases, these additional operations are performed for specific indications related to coexisting disease processes. More often, however, this additional surgery is performed for prophylactic reasons. In an extensive review by Dicker et al,[1] 79.5% of women undergoing abdominal hysterectomy and 62.0% of women undergoing vaginal hysterectomy had concurrent surgical procedures. In the majority of cases, these were gynecologic operations (Table 8.1).

When planning concomitant surgery during hysterectomy, several important considerations must be made. Will the additional procedure add significant intraoperative and postoperative morbidity? Do the benefits of performing the additional operation outweigh the operative risks to the patient and the later risks incurred if this procedure is not performed? This is an especially important consideration when planning prophylactic surgery. Finally, does performing a hysterectomy effect the success of an additional operative procedure, and does it increase any associated morbidity? Weighing all of these factors allows the surgeon to develop a precise and individualized surgical plan for each patient. In addition, the patient is well informed of her alternatives, allowing her to knowledgeably participate in the ultimate decision for her care.

Oophorectomy

Bilateral oophorectomy is the most common concurrent operation performed at the time of hysterectomy. In most cases, it is a prophylactic procedure involving the removal of grossly and histologically normal ovaries. No consensus opinion exists as to the indications and timing for oophorectomy. Proposed reasons for the removal of normal ovaries include prevention of ovarian cancer later in life, avoiding reoperation

Table 8.1 Concurrent Surgical Procedures Among Women Ages 15 to 44 Undergoing Hysterectomy, by Surgical Approach, CREST,[a] 1978 to 1981

Procedure	Vaginal ($n = 568$)	Abdominal ($n = 1,283$)	Total ($N = 1,851$)
Any concurrent procedure (%)	62.0	79.5	74.1
Adnexal surgery (%)	7.6	57.6	42.2
Colporrhaphy (%)	44.5	0.8	14.2
Appendectomy (%)	0	17.5	12.1
Urethral suspension (%)	0.5	2.7	2.1

[a] CREST, Collaborative Review of Sterilization.
Reprinted, by permission, from Dicker RC, Greenspan JR, Strauss LT, et al: Complications of abdominal and vaginal hysterectomy among women of reproductive age in the United States. Am J Obstet Gynecol 1982;144:841–848.

secondary to the development of benign adnexal pathology, and, in rare cases, the alleviation of symptoms of severe premenstrual syndrome. Opponents of oophorectomy contend that the risks of ovarian cancer after hysterectomy are minimal and that the incidence of cancer would not be greatly affected by this routine surgical practice. They also state that hormone replacement therapy cannot completely simulate the natural production and effects of sex steroids, and that oophorectomy can lead to significant psychological disturbances.

Pokras and Hufnagel[2] found that from 1965 to 1984, the incidence of oophorectomy at the time of hysterectomy rose from 25% to 41%. Dicker et al[1] found a similar incidence of 42.2% when reviewing 1,851 women undergoing hysterectomy between 1978 and 1981. When analyzed by age of the patient, over a 25-year period the overall incidence of oophorectomy at the time of hysterectomy was 36% for patients 39 years of age or younger, 41% for those 40 to 49, and 48% for patients 50 years of age or older.[3] An interesting study in Great Britain submitted questionnaires to members and fellows of the Royal College of Obstetricians and Gynaecologists, asking about their practice of routine oophorectomy at the time of hysterectomy.[4] The percentage of respondents who removed normal ovaries during abdominal hysterectomy in premenopausal women in age groups 35 to 59, 40 to 44, 45 to 49, and over 49 years was 0.4%, 2%, 20%, and 51%, respectively, and in postmenopausal women was 85%.

With a mean incidence for routine oophorectomy approximating 42% and a projected 810,000 hysterectomies performed annually by 1995, a significant number of women will have normal ovaries removed.[2] Although the majority of these women will be postmenopausal, a large number will be premenopausal and over 45 years of age. The continued functioning of ovaries in these women, and subsequent function once menopause is reached, are important concepts to understand when planning concommitant oophorectomy. When assessing 92 women under 50 years of age who previously underwent hysterectomy with the preservation of one or both ovaries, DeNeef and Hollenbeck[5] reported that vaginal cytology in 89 women demonstrated estrogen production and that only three patients definitely had a menopausal smear. Randall et al[6] and coworkers have shown that only 13% of patients having a hysterectomy with preservation of the ovaries showed evidence of ovarian deficiency when examined 2 to 5 years after their surgery. In addition, only 29.3% of the women followed 10 to 15 years after hysterectomy with ovarian preservation demonstrated ovarian deficiency. In the same study, over 4% of women examined 10 to 15 years after natural cessation of menses showed definite estrogen effect. Obviously, ovarian function continues with significant estrogen effect into the early 50s, with the mean age for menopause being approximately 52 years. Removal of the ovaries at age 45 or younger would rob the patient of 7 to 10 years of cyclic estrogen production. In addition, postmenopausal ovarian steroid production plays a role in estrogen availability through peripheral conversion of androstenedione. Although production is lower than in the premenopausal state, this androgen release may play a significant functional role not only in health maintenance of the patient but in her overall well-being.

Advantages of Oophorectomy

The primary advantage and the most common indication for prophylactic oophorectomy at the time of hysterectomy is the prevention of ovarian cancer later in life. The lifetime risk of developing ovarian cancer has been quoted as from 0.9% to 1.4%.[7,8] Diagnosis is rarely made in early-stage disease, with the overall 5-year survival at only 37%.[8] With no reliable method of early detection available, the impetus for prophylactic removal of the ovaries during hysterectomy is strong. Data reporting the impact of prophylactic oophorectomy on the incidence of ovarian cancer are controversial, and in most cases estimations. Several reports have suggested that routine oophorectomy at the time of hysterectomy could lower the incidence of cancer by 10% to 12%.[4,9,10] This would correlate to a small reduction in the incidence from 9/1,000 women to 8/1,000 women. Hysterectomy with ovarian preservation does not appear to increase the risk for cancer of the ovary. In fact, just the opposite association has been found. Annegers et al[11] showed a 5% incidence of prior hysterectomy in ovarian cancer patients compared to a 23% incidence of hysterectomy for matched controls. Counseller et al[12] demonstrated similar results. However, when reviewing patients who had undergone a hysterectomy greater than 10 years earlier, Weiss and Harlow[13] found the relative risk for developing ovarian cancer was 1.6. In light of the other studies, this small increase in risk is questionable. Further prospective analysis of the effect of hysterectomy on the development of ovarian cancer is necessary. Finally, prophylactic oophorectomy may not completely prevent ovarian cancer in women of cancer-prone families. Tobacman et al[14] found that, when prophylactic oophorectomy was performed in 28 female members of 16 cancer-prone families, three of the women developed disseminated intraabdominal malignancy histopathologically indistinguishable from ovarian carcinoma. Genetic predisposition to multicentric neoplasia from celomic epithelium was proposed to account for the development of cancer in these women.

The incidence of reoperation for benign ovarian and/or adnexal disease following hysterectomy with preservation of one or both ovaries ranges between 2.4% and 5%.[15-17] DeNeef and Hollenbeck[5] reported that four of seven patients requiring reoperation for removal of the ovaries had their surgery within 1 year of their hysterectomy. In the majority of cases, an adnexal mass, pelvic pain, and dyspareunia are presenting symptoms that lead the patient to reoperation. Grogan,[17] in his reappraisal of the residual ovary, suggested that previous conservative pelvic surgery prior to hysterectomy, and dysfunctional ovaries associated with abnormal uterine bleeding, may be associated risk factors for later oophorectomy after hysterectomy. Few data exist to confirm these statements. Finally, removal of the ovaries at the time of hysterectomy is not a guarantee that ovarian disease will not develop later. Symmonds and Pettit[16] reviewed 20 cases of ovarian remnant syndrome, stating that this entity represented a complication of a difficult oophorectomy. Predisposing factors to the development of ovarian remnant syndrome were the presence of pelvic inflammatory disease, endometriosis, and dense pelvic adhesions. In summary, the risk of benign ovarian pathology developing after hysterectomy is minimal and unpredictable, and should therefore not affect the decision to remove both ovaries.

Alleviation of severe premenstrual syndrome by oophorectomy combined with hysterectomy has received attention within the last 5 to 10 years. Casper and Hearn[18] reported a series of 14 patients who underwent abdominal hysterectomy with bilateral salpingo-oophorectomy, followed by estrogen replacement therapy, for the treatment of severe premenstrual syndrome unresponsive to conservative therapy. Resolution of premenstrual symptoms was noted in all patients. Scores for general affect, well-being, and quality of life were essentially equal to those of a matched group of normal patients. Casson and coworkers[19] administered danazol to 14 patients with severe premenstrual syndrome, suppressing cyclic ovarian function and premenstrual symptoms. When their severe symptoms returned following discontinuation of the drug, all 14 patients opted for bilateral ovariectomy with hysterectomy, resulting in a return to their asymptomatic state. Both of these studies, although showing good results with bilateral oophorectomy when treating severe premenstrual syndrome, consisted of small groups of patients who were all volunteers. In addition, no matched controls were utilized. As noted by Casson et al,[19] surgical treatment for premenstrual syndrome should be considered only as a last resort for a carefully screened group of patients. Further prospective analysis of this practice is necessary to judge its proper utilization for a very select group of patients.

Disadvantages of Oophorectomy

The disadvantages of oophorectomy at the time of hysterectomy, especially in premenopausal women, are those related to the absence of endogenous sex steroid production. The practice of countering these effects with hormone replacement therapy is argued against by those who state that normal hormone production is poorly simulated by exogenous sources. Menopausal symptoms, osteoporosis, cardiovascular disease, and various psychological stigmata are often inadequately relieved.

The onset of menopausal symptoms following surgical ablation of the ovaries is an extremely distressing problem. Symptoms are often more strongly manifested and more difficult to control when compared with natural menopause. DeNeef and Hollenbeck[5] noted the onset of hot flushes, depression, and irritability in 52.2% of patients undergoing bilateral oophorectomy at the time of hysterectomy. However, when analyzing other women in the study undergoing hysterectomy, 35.6% with both ovaries remaining and 34.8% with one ovary remaining were noted to complain of menopausal symptoms. Obviously removal of the ovaries, and the subsequent fall in serum estrogen levels, leads to these disturbing symptoms. However, the uterus may play a role in controlling menopausal symptomatology through the direct action of uterine secretions such as prostaglandins or through indirect control by balancing cyclic ovarian activity, as evidenced by DeNeef and Hollenbeck's study.[5,20]

Numerous hormone replacement regimens have been described to alleviate constitutional symptoms, and the clinical and metabolic alterations occurring as a result of surgical menopause. The ability to closely reproduce premenopausal steroid hormone balance is the primary goal of each regimen. However, this is never completely possible. Studies have shown that gonadotropin levels rise approximately 2 days after oophorectomy and cannot be adequately reduced by standard estrogen replacement therapy.[21,22] When studying 11 surgically menopausal patients, Utian et al[21] demonstrated small reductions in serum follicle-stimulating hormone (FSH) with standard oral doses of conjugated estrogens. Premenopausal levels of FSH were achieved in only one instance by producing a hyperestrogenic state with doses of 2.5 mg/day. Even with excessive doses of estrogen, luteinizing hormone (LH) levels were not lowered out of postmenopausal ranges. Although normal estradiol serum levels were obtained with standard daily doses of 0.625 mg and 1.25 mg, the benefit in light of elevated gonadotropins, and the importance of achieving premenopausal sex hormone profiles, still remain questionable.

Bilateral ovariectomy in the premenopausal patient may have a significant impact on bone loss and the incidence of osteoporosis. Hreshchyshyn et al[23] have shown significantly lower bone densities in premenopausally oophorectomized patients when compared to patients who went through natural menopause, patients who had postmenopausal oophorectomy, and patients who had a hysterectomy without oophorectomy. These differences were maintained whether or not the premenopausal patients who had an oophorectomy were receiving hormone replacement therapy. It is theorized that the abrupt removal of estrogen by oophorectomy accounts for a rapid diminution in bone density, especially since postmenopausal oophorectomy does not affect bone density. The administration of estrogen replacement therapy partially restores lumbar bone density, but does not reach density values measured in those patients going through natural menopause or having a hysterectomy only—an effect that cannot be fully explained.[23]

In addition to a precipitous fall in serum estrogen levels after surgical removal of the ovaries, a decrease in testosterone levels also occurs. The reduction of this hormone, and other androgens, is believed to play a significant role in altering certain psychological parameters and sexual behavior in premenopausal women. When comparing surgically menopausal women who received an estrogen-androgen combination or androgen alone to those who received estrogen alone or placebo, Sherwin and Gelfand[24] found a statistically significant improvement in energy level, appetite, and overall well-being. In addition, similar improvements in the sexual parameters of desire, arousal, fantasies, and rates of coitus and orgasm were seen in surgically menopausal women receiving an estrogen-androgen combination when compared to those receiving estrogen alone or placebo.[25]

Technique of Oophorectomy at Vaginal Hysterectomy

From a technical standpoint, the surgical procedure of bilateral oophorectomy or salpingo-oophorectomy has been thoroughly described in most major gynecologic surgery textbooks. However, because most oophorectomies are performed at the time of abdominal hysterectomy, removal of the ovaries at the time of vaginal hysterectomy, and a description of its concomitant complications, has strangely received little attention. In one of the largest series available, Smale et al[26] reviewed 355 patients undergoing vaginal hysterectomy with removal of the adnexa. No differences were found in length of hospital stay and febrile morbidity between patients who had bilateral oophorectomy and those who had vaginal hysterectomy alone. Only one patient required laparotomy for control of bleeding from the ovarian pedicle. Injury to the ureter has been cited as a major risk when performing vaginal adnexectomy. Radiologic studies by Hofmeister and Wolfgram[27] have shown that, when clamping the infundibulopelvic ligaments, the ureters are only 2 cm from the clamps. In neither Smale et al's study[26] nor a review of 77 patients by Capen et al[28] was an injury to the ureter incurred. Obviously, meticulous surgical technique and careful attention to anatomic relationships are necessary in order to avoid this complication. In one of the only prospective analyses of the ability to remove the adnexa vaginally, Hoffman[29] used a combination of clamp techniques and endoscopic loop suture to remove 31 of 40 ovaries (77.5%) in 20 patients undergoing vaginal hysterectomy. Although a paucity of data exist on the rates of removing ovaries through the vagina, anecdotally 60% to 70% is the reported incidence.[28]

Summary

Removal of the ovaries at the time of hysterectomy requires individualized comparison of the advantages and disadvantages. Although the incidence of ovarian cancer and the development of benign adnexal pathology after hysterectomy alone is extremely small, the development of either should be avoided. In most cases, symptomatic relief of surgical menopause can be achieved with hormone replacement therapy, but many clinical and metabolic parameters lack perfect return to their premenopausal states. In general, selecting an arbitrary age for removal of the ovaries is not practical. However, keeping all of the information reviewed in perspective, postmenopausal removal of the ovaries at the time of hysterectomy should be an acceptable practice.

Colporrhaphy and Management of the Vaginal Vault

Between 1978 and 1981, Dicker et al[1] found the incidence of colporrhaphy at the time of vaginal hysterectomy to be 44.5%. The most important consideration prior to performing a colporrhaphy or vaginal vault supportive procedure at the time of hysterectomy is whether or not the additional procedure is truly indicated. Once determined, the question of additional risk should be answered. Risks of operative and postoperative morbidity from a vaginal plastic procedure must be considered, as well as intrinsic risks to the additional operation by combining it with a vaginal hysterectomy.

Classically, indications for anterior colporrhaphy include the correction of symptomatic cystocele and mild to moderate stress urinary incontinence. Although retropubic urethropexy has essentially replaced anterior colporrhaphy as the standard surgical treatment for stress incontinence, the anterior vaginal approach is still widely utilized. In general, correction rates for stress incontinence of 60% to 65% can be expected, with rates as high as 94% quoted by some.[30] Posterior colporrhaphy is indicated for the surgical correction of a symptomatic rectocele, and in some instances a relaxed vaginal outlet. In most cases, however, a simple perineal repair is all that is necessary for relaxation of the outer vagina.[31]

Several studies have addressed the issues of additional intraoperative and postoperative morbidity when performing anterior and posterior colporrhaphy at the time of vaginal hysterectomy. When comparing patients who underwent vaginal hysterectomy and salpingo-oophorectomy to patients having the same operations with an anterior and/or posterior colporrhaphy, Capen et al[28] found the average drop in postoperative hematocrit was only 1.9% greater in the latter group. In addition, this study and a review by Dicker et al[1] found no increase in the rate of postoperative fever when colporrhaphies were performed. Dicker et al's study found that the average hospital stay for women having a vaginal hysterectomy was 5 days, and for those having a vaginal hysterectomy with colporrhaphy it was 6 days. To investigate the influence of age on the incidence of morbidity associated with vaginal hysterectomy combined with anterior and posterior colporrhaphy, Taylor and Hansen[32] compared a group of women 35 years of age or younger to a group of women 50 years of age or older. Their findings revealed a significantly higher incidence of prolonged operating time, blood replacement, febrile morbidity, prolonged convalescence, and pelvic hematoma or abscess in the younger patients. These findings were believed to be the result of greater vascularity in the younger group. The study failed to note if there was a difference in the degree of pelvic relaxation between younger and older patients, a factor possibly leading to a more difficult procedure in younger patients who might lack significant defects.

The addition of anterior colporrhaphy to vaginal hysterectomy has been claimed to lead to various forms of lower urinary tract dysfunction.[1,33] Dicker et al[1] noted that, whereas urinary retention occurred in 8% of women undergoing vaginal hysterectomy alone, the addition of an anterior colporrhaphy was associated with retention in 24% of the patients. In contrast, Stanton et al[34] prospectively evaluated 73 patients undergoing anterior colporrhaphy, 46 of whom also had a vaginal hysterectomy, and found no increase in the incidence of voiding dysfunction and detrusor instability within or between the two groups. Although all patients in this study had good correction of their anterior vaginal relaxation, 20 of 29 patients having a preoperative diagnosis of stress urinary incontinence were still incontinent after surgery. In addition, five patients who were continent prior to surgery developed stress incontinence postoperatively, two with anterior repair alone and three with anterior repair and vaginal hysterectomy.

The use of various additional surgical techniques for managing the vaginal vault at the time of vaginal hysterectomy generates significant controversy. The addition of these procedures is recommended either to avoid the development of a postoperative enterocele or to prevent posthysterectomy vaginal vault prolapse. Standard surgical management of the vaginal vault has described variations of peritoneal closure techniques that incorporate attachment and plication of the uterosacral and cardinal ligament pedicles.[35–37] However, culdoplasty techniques, such as those described by McCall[38] and Torpin,[39] are frequently added to a vaginal hysterectomy in order to prevent enterocele formation at a later time. In addition to the culdoplasties, others have recommended the use of sacrospinous vaginal vault suspension at the time of vaginal hysterectomy to prevent vault prolapse in women thought to be at risk for this complication.[40]

Although culdoplasty techniques are recommended to prevent posthysterectomy enterocele formation, no precise objective predictors have been identified to show who is at risk for enterocele development. Logically, one would assume that the presence of a lax posterior cul-de-sac or moderate to severe uterine descensus could eventually lead to an enterocele after hysterectomy. Since 1956, surgeons at the Mayo Clinic have routinely performed prophylactic culdoplasty with vaginal hysterectomy, providing the clinical impression that vault prolapse or enterocele may be prevented later.[41] In one of the only prospective studies evaluating the success of culdoplasty techniques, Given[42] operated on 68 patients, 18 of whom were having a vaginal hysterectomy for uterine procidentia. Of these 18 cases, two failures were noted during follow-up. In addition to surgical failures, rare complications of culdoplasties have included vaginal shortening, dyspareunia, nerve palsy, and ureteral obstruction.[41,42]

Cruikshank and Cox performed prophylactic sacrospinous fixation of the vagina in 48 of 135 patients undergoing vaginal hysterectomy.[40] These 48 patients were thought to be "at risk" for later vaginal vault prolapse because they demonstrated moderate to severe uterovaginal prolapse. During a follow-up of 8 months to 3.2 years, no vaginal vault prolapse occurred in these women. Although this prophylactic procedure was successful and complications were minimal, several points must be considered. The incidence of posthysterectomy vaginal vault prolapse is approximately 0.2%.[41] Therefore, as Morley's discussion of Cruikshank's article[43] has pointed out, it would take over 200 patients undergoing this prophylactic procedure to prevent one vault prolapse. Both Symmonds et al[41] and Given[42] found that only 39% and 42%, respectively, of posthysterectomy vault prolapses were noted at 2 years of follow-up. Therefore a much longer follow-up of patients will be necessary to assess the prophylactic use of sacrospinous vault suspension. Finally, there are no data to support the contention that moderate to severe uterovaginal prolapse is a risk for later posthysterectomy vaginal vault prolapse. A randomized comparative study within this group of patients would be necessary to prove that point and answer whether this prophylactic operation is of value for moderate to severe prolapse.

Pelvic relaxation is the most common indication for vaginal hysterectomy.[1] Because accompanying defects will be present, surgical methods for managing them, especially the vaginal vault, will be necessary. When little relaxation is present, simple closure of the cuff with attachment or plication of the pedicles is probably all that is necessary. For moderate to severe prolapse, one of the various culdoplasty techniques may be advisable. In light of failures with culdoplasties when procidentia is present, an accompanying sacrospinous fixation may be indicated.

Incontinence Surgery: Retropubic Urethropexy

In general, the transabdominal retropubic approach to incontinence surgery has become the most common and successful operative route. A long-held dictum in gynecologic surgical teaching has been that, when performing a retropubic urethropexy for stress urinary incontinence, a concomitant hysterectomy should also be performed to improve the results.[44] More recently, this view has been challenged. A review of the effects of hysterectomy on urinary function is indicated, as well as assessing the objective contribution to restoring urinary control in women with urodynamically proven stress urinary incontinence.

Several studies have examined the effects of hysterectomy on urinary function. Parys et al[45] evaluated preoperative and postoperative urinary function and sacral reflex latencies in 36 women undergoing simple hysterectomy for benign disease. New urodynamic abnormalities were noted in 11/36 women (30.6%) postoperatively, with 38.9% demonstrating abnormal studies prior to surgery. Of the 11 new abnormalities, five were genuine stress incontinence, three urethral obstruction, two detrusor instability, and one genuine stress incontinence with urethral obstruction. Eleven women showed evidence of pelvic nerve neuropathy, and eight of these also had altered vesicourethral dysfunction. Langer et al[46] evaluated 16 premenopausal women lacking urinary symptoms who underwent total abdominal hysterectomy for benign conditions. Contrary to Parys et al's study,[45] no symptoms of frequency, urgency, urge, or stress incontinence were noted postoperatively. In addition, no alteration in values from cystometry, uroflowmetry, or urethral pressure profilometry occurred after hysterectomy.

To assess the effect of hysterectomy on the successful correction of stress incontinence with a Burch retropubic urethropexy, Sand et al[47] retrospectively reviewed results in 86 women undergoing the Burch colposuspension, in 62 of whom a hysterectomy had also been performed. A failure rate of 42% was noted in the group who had previously had a hysterectomy, as compared to a failure rate of only 17% in patients maintaining their uterus. In a prospective randomized comparative study, Langer et al[48] evaluated the effect of concomitant hysterectomy by following 22 women who had a Burch colposuspension alone and 23 women who had a colposuspension combined with total abdominal hysterectomy and cul-de-sac obliteration. All 45 patients in the study had no uterine disease or significant pelvic floor defects preoperatively. Cure rates for stress incontinence were almost identical between the two groups when objective testing was performed (95.5% for the no-hysterectomy group and 95.7% for the hysterectomy group). These findings are similar to those of Stanton and Cardozo,[49] who evaluated 88 patients 1 year after Burch colposuspension, demonstrating no differences in cure rates between 43 patients who had a hysterectomy and 45 patients who did not. In Langer et al's study,[48] although there was no difference in the incidence of intraoperative or immediate postoperative complications, three women (13.5%) in the no-hysterectomy group developed a postoperative enterocele, whereas no one in the other group developed this anatomic defect.

In summary, there is little recent objective evidence to support the belief that performing a hysterectomy is necessary when a retropubic urethropexy is performed for the treatment of genuine stress incontinence. In fact, hysterectomy may be detrimental to the desired results. Additional long-term follow-up studies are needed to resolve this issue. In general, a hysterectomy is indicated at the time of retropubic cystourethropexy only when a concomitant gynecologic indication dictates its necessity.

Appendectomy

Reasons for performing incidental appendectomy at the time of hysterectomy include preventing appendicitis, either later in life or in the immediate postoperative period, and removing undiagnosed pathology in the appendix. Opposition to routine removal of a normal-appearing appendix addresses concerns of potential increases in intraoperative and postoperative morbidity.

The true incidence of appendicitis is unknown. It is most common in the second and third decades of life, a period far before the average age at which hysterectomy is most commonly performed.[50] When the appendix has been removed, the differential diagnosis of appendicitis can be excluded in the woman who presents with acute lower abdominal and pelvic pain.

Microscopic abnormalities in normal appendices removed at the time of hysterectomy are quite common. Whether these histopathologic findings eventually lead to clinical morbidity is unknown. Melcher[51] noted that only 12 of 45 appendices incidentally removed at the time of hysterectomy were microscopically normal. In two cases, asymptomatic carcinoid tumors were found. In a review of 830 appendectomies performed at the time of hysterectomy, Waters[52] found that 22% of the cases revealed pathologic alterations significant enough to warrant removal of a grossly normal-appearing appendix. Five carcinoid tumors were found in this study.

Several large retrospective studies have reviewed the incidence of intraoperative and postoperative morbidity when incidental appendectomy has been combined with abdominal hysterectomy.[52–54] In each of these studies, a similar group of patients who underwent hysterectomy alone was used for comparison. In none of these investigations was a significant difference in febrile morbidity, requirement for antibiotics, wound infection, blood loss, or length of hospital stay demonstrated. One interesting finding by Loeffler and Stearn[53] showed that, whereas no patient having an appendectomy developed a postoperative ileus or obstruction, this complication occurred in four patients who had a hysterectomy alone. Voitk and Lowry[54] analyzed the additional operating time for an appendectomy and found the average to be 10 minutes.

In general, the addition of appendectomy at the time of abdominal hysterectomy does not increase morbidity or mortality. In experienced hands it appears to be a safe, if not advisable, practice as a means of prophylaxis against appendicitis and the possible development of appendiceal pathology. Although few data exist to support its practice, of note is a report by McGowan[55] in which he performed 10 appendectomies by the vaginal route, eight with vaginal hysterectomy incurring no additional blood loss or fever.

Cholecystectomy

Gallbladder disease occurs most often in the fifth and sixth decades of life, and is four times more common in women than men.[56,57] Because the fifth decade of life is the most common age range for hysterectomy, it is not unusual that a woman who has indications for a hysterectomy also has disease of the gallbladder, specifically cholelithiasis. Combining hysterectomy and cholescystectomy is common practice around the country, with the impetus being to save the patient from undergoing two anesthesias. The possibility of increased intraoperative and postoperative morbidity is the greatest detractor from this combination procedure.

Both Pratt et al[56] and Murray et al[57] reviewed 95 and 21 patients, respectively, who underwent combination hysterectomy and cholecystectomy. All of Murray et al's patients had abdominal hysterectomies, whereas 67 of Pratt et al's patients had abdominal hysterectomies and 28 had vaginal hysterectomies. In neither study was there a significant increase in postoperative febrile morbidity or length of hospital stay when compared to similar patients having hysterectomy alone. Whereas 19% of the patients in Murray et al's study required blood transfusion, Pratt et al found transfusions necessary in 65.5% of patients having vaginal hysterectomy and in 18.6% having abdominal hysterectomy. Mean operating time in Murray et al's study was 3.3 hours. Postoperative ileus occurred infrequently in both studies and was not different from incidences noted when the operations were performed individually. Pratt et al noted two deaths in their group of 95 patients, both resulting from coronary occlusion. One patient died 11 days postoperatively. The other died intraoperatively, possibly related to excessive blood loss during vaginal hysterectomy and a tenuous cardiovascular status related to age.

Although some drawbacks of combination hysterectomy-cholecystectomy have been noted, the results achieved when patients are carefully chosen are usually satisfactory. For older patients with significant medical illnesses, potential prolonged operating time and the need for blood replacement should be considered. In the middle-aged healthy woman, this combination approach has attractive advantages.

Abdominoplasty and Liposuction

Abdominoplasty is described as a lower abdominal lipectomy combined with musculofascial repair.[58] Indications for this procedure are cosmetic and include abdominal obesity, dermatochalasis (lax skin), or a combination of the two.[59] The most common complications described with abdominoplasty have been wound infection and breakdown, skin necrosis, injury to the lateral cutaneous nerve of the thigh, hematoma, and pulmonary embolus.[58–60] The procedure is most commonly performed in women between the ages 35 and 40 years, and it is becoming increasingly popular for women to request this elective plastic operation at the time of an indicated hysterectomy.[59,60]

Several studies have examined the safety of performing abdominoplasty at the time of hysterectomy. Voss et al[60] compared the outcomes of three groups of patients: those undergoing a gynecologic procedure and abdominoplasty ($n = 76$), those undergoing a gynecologic procedure alone ($n = 76$), and those undergoing an abdominoplasty alone ($n = 70$). The combination procedure resulted in a shorter hospital stay, shorter operating time, and lower intraoperative blood loss than the sum of the means from the two singular operations. The combination did not result in lower postoperative blood loss, and this group required more transfusions. Five patients in the combination group suffered pulmonary emboli after surgery, whereas no women in either of the single-operation groups experienced this complication. Weight over 70 kg and age over 50 years were considered to be risks for a pulmonary embolus when gynecologic surgery (especially abdominal hysterectomy) was combined with an abdominoplasty. In a similar study, Hester et al[58] compared patients having abdominoplasty alone to patients having abdominoplasty combined with pelvic surgery or abdominoplasty combined with another aesthetic procedure (usually mammoplasty). There was a higher incidence of transfusion in the combination groups, but there was no difference in the infection rates. Again, pulmonary embolus occurred at a higher rate when combination procedures were performed. Whereas there were no pulmonary emboli in the abdominoplasty group, 4/230 women in the abdominoplasty and gynecologic procedure group experienced an embolus. Although age did not appear to be a risk in this study, obesity was again significantly associated with the occurrence of pulmonary emboli.

One study has examined the feasibility and safety of combining liposuction with hysterectomy. Kovac[61] prospectively compared 50 women undergoing vaginal hysterectomy with a matched group of 50 women undergoing vaginal hysterectomy combined with liposuction of the abdomen, buttocks, and thighs. There was no difference between groups with regard to hospital stay. Eight patients in the vaginal hysterectomy group developed fever compared to four in the combination group. Only two patients required transfusion, both of whom had liposuction of more than 2,000 mL of fat.

It is apparent that combining aesthetic abdominal procedures with hysterectomy can reduce hospital stay and save an extra anesthetic experience when compared with both operations performed separately. However, this must be balanced with the greater risk for transfusion and the potential risk of pulmonary embolus. For the young, healthy woman, careful planning of combination abdominoplasty and hysterectomy is acceptable. However, for the obese woman over 50 years of age, separate procedures seem advisable. Combining liposuction with hysterectomy appears to involve less risk, especially when fat removal is less than 2,000 mL. Further study in this area is necessary.

Conclusion

Above all, the most important consideration when planning concomitant surgery with a hysterectomy is whether the procedure is truly indicated. The advantages and disadvantages of the additional operation should be carefully weighed. The procedure cannot be lightly undertaken, based on anecdotal past experience or the desire to "kill two birds with one stone." As newer surgical techniques are introduced, especially endoscopic procedures, increased utilization of combination operations may occur. As with all new surgical techniques, prospective comparative trials are necessary to prove their value for the patient and the surgeon.

References

1. Dicker RC, Greenspan JR, Strauss LT, et al: Complications of abdominal and vaginal hysterectomy among women of reproductive age in the United States. *Am J Obstet Gynecol* 1982;144:841–848.
2. Pokras R, Hufnagel VG: Hysterectomy in the United States, 1965–84. *Am J Public Health* 1988;78:852–853.
3. Randall CL, Paloucek FP: The frequency of oophorectomy at the time of hysterectomy. *Am J Obstet Gynecol* 1968;100:716–726.
4. Jacobs I, Oram D: Prevention of ovarian cancer: A survey of the practice of prophylactic oophorectomy by fellows and members of the Royal College of Obstetricians and Gynaecologists. *Br J Obstet Gynaecol* 1989;96:510–515.
5. DeNeef JC, Hollenbeck ZJR: The fate of the ovaries preserved at the time of hysterectomy. *Am J Obstet Gynecol* 1966;96:1088–1097.
6. Randall CL, Birtch PK, Harkins JL: Ovarian function after menopause. *Am J Obstet Gynecol* 1957;74:719–729.
7. Randall CL, Gerhardt PR: The probability of the occurrence of the more common types of gynecologic malignancy. *Am J Obstet Gynecol* 1954;68:1378–1390.
8. Barber HRK: Ovarian cancer. *Cancer* 1986;36:149–184.
9. Howe HL: Age-specific hysterectomy and oophorectomy prevalence rates and the risk for cancer of the reproductive system. *Am J Public Health* 1984;74:560–563.

10. Grundsell H, Ekman G, Gullberg B, et al: Some aspects of prophylactic oophorectomy and ovarian carcinoma. *Ann Chir Gynaecol* 1981;70:36–42.
11. Annegers JF, Strom H, Decker DG, et al: Ovarian cancer: Incidence and case-control study. *Cancer* 1979;43:723–729.
12. Counseller VS, Hunt W, Haigler FH: Carcinoma of the ovary following hysterectomy. *Am J Obstet Gynecol* 1955;69:538–546.
13. Weiss NS, Harlow BL: Why does hysterectomy without bilateral oophorectomy influence the subsequent incidence of ovarian cancer? *Am J Epidemiol* 1986;124:856–858.
14. Tobacman JK, Tucker MA, Kase R, et al: Intra-abdominal carcinomatosis after prophylactic oophorectomy in ovarian-cancer-prone families. *Lancet* 1982;2:795–797.
15. Loizzi P, Carriero C, DiGesie A, et al: Removal or preservation of ovaries during hysterectomy: A six year review. *Int J Gynecol Obstet* 1990;31:257–261.
16. Symmonds RE, Pettit PDM: Ovarian remnant syndrome. *Obstet Gynecol* 1979;54:174–177.
17. Grogan RH: Reappraisal of residual ovaries. *Am J Obstet Gynecol* 1967;97:124–129.
18. Casper RF, Hearn MT: The effect of hysterectomy and bilateral oophorectomy in women with severe premenstrual syndrome. *Am J Obstet Gynecol* 1990;162:105–109.
19. Casson P, Hahn PM, Van Vugt DA, et al: Lasting response to ovariectomy in severe intractable premenstrual syndrome. *Am J Obstet Gynecol* 1990;162:99–105.
20. Garcia C, Cutler WB: Preservation of the ovary: A reevaluation. *Fertil Steril* 1984;42:510–514.
21. Utian WH, Katz M, Davey DA, et al: Effect of premenstrual castration and incremental doses of conjugated equine estrogens on plasma follicle-stimulating hormone, luteinizing hormone, and estradiol. *Am J Obstet Gynecol* 1978;132:297–302.
22. Wallach EE, Root AW, Garcia C: Serum gonadotropin responses to estrogen and progestin in recently castrated human females. *J Clin Endocrinol Metab* 1970;31:376–381.
23. Hreshchyshyn MM, Hopkins A, Zylstra S, et al: Effects of natural menopause, hysterectomy, and oophorectomy on lumbar spine and femoral neck bone densities. *Obstet Gynecol* 1988;72:631–638.
24. Sherwin BB, Gelfand MM: Differential symptom response to parenteral estrogen and/or androgen administration in the surgical menopause. *Am J Obstet Gynecol* 1985;151:153–160.
25. Sherwin BB, Gelfand MM: The role of androgen in the maintenance of sexual functioning in oophorectomized women. *Psychosom Med* 1987;49:397–409.
26. Smale LE, Smale ML, Wilkening RL, et al: Salpingo-oophorectomy at the time of vaginal hysterectomy. *Am J Obstet Gynecol* 1978;131:122–128.
27. Hofmeister FJ, Wolfgram RC: Methods of demonstrating measurement relationships between vaginal hysterectomy ligatures and the ureters. *Am J Obstet Gynecol* 1962;83:938–948.
28. Cape CV, Irwin H, Magrina J, et al: Vaginal removal of the ovaries in association with vaginal hysterectomy. *J Reprod Med* 1983;28:589–591.

29. Hoffman MS: Transvaginal removal of ovaries with Endoloop suture at the time of transvaginal hysterectomy. *Am J Obstet Gynecol* 1991;165:407–408.
30. Beck RP, McCormick S, Nordstrom L: A 25 year experience with 519 anterior colporrhaphy procedures. *Obstet Gynecol* 1991;78:1011–1018.
31. Thompson JD: Relaxed vaginal outlet, rectocele, fecal incontinence, and rectovaginal fistula, in Thompson JD, Rock JA (eds): *TeLinde's Operative Gynecology*, ed 7. Philadelphia, JB Lippincott, 1992, pp 941–978.
32. Taylor ES, Hansen RR: Morbidity following vaginal hysterectomy and culdoplasty. *Obstet Gynecol* 1961;17:346–348.
33. Tanagho EA: Effects of hysterectomy and pariurethral surgery on urethrovesical function, in Ostergard DR (ed): *Gynecologic Urology and Urodynamics: Theory and Practice*, ed 2. Baltimore, Williams & Wilkins, 1985, pp 537–544.
34. Stanton SL, Norton C, Cardozo L: Clinical and urodynamic effects of anterior colporrhaphy and vaginal hysterectomy for prolapse with or without incontinence. *Br J Obstet Gynaecol* 1982;89:459–463.
35. Thompson JD: Hysterectomy, in Thompson JD, Rock JA (eds): *TeLinde's Operative Gynecology*, ed 7. Philadelphia, JB Lippincott, 1992, pp 663–738.
36. Hajj SN: A simplified surgical technique for the treatment of the vault in vaginal hysterectomy. *Am J Obstet Gynecol* 1979;133:851–854.
37. Cruikshank SH: Preventing posthysterectomy vaginal vault prolapse and enterocele during vaginal hysterectomy. *Am J Obstet Gynecol* 1987;156:1433–1440.
38. McCall ML: Posterior culdoplasty: Surgical correction of enterocele during vaginal hysterectomy; a preliminary report. *Obstet Gynecol* 1957;10:595–602.
39. Torpin R: Excision of the cul-de-sac of Douglas: For the surgical cure of hernias, through the female caudal wall, including prolapse of the uterus. *J Int Coll Surg* 1955;24:322–330.
40. Cruikshank SH, Cox DW: Sacrospinous ligament fixation at the time of transvaginal hysterectomy. *Am J Obstet Gynecol* 1990;162:1611–1619.
41. Symmonds RE, Williams TJ, Lee TJ, et al: Posthysterectomy enterocele and vaginal vault prolapse. *Am J Obstet Gynecol* 1981;140:852–859.
42. Given FT: Posterior culdeplasty: Revisited. *Am J Obstet Gynecol* 1985;153:135–139.
43. Morley GW, DeLancey JOL: Sacrospinous ligament fixation for eversion of the vagina. *Am J Obstet Gynecol* 1988;158:872–881.
44. Green TH: Urinary stress incontinence: Differential diagnosis, pathophysiology, and management. *Am J Obstet Gynecol* 1975;122:368–400.
45. Parys BT, Haylen BT, Hutton JL, et al: The effects of simple hysterectomy on vesicourethral function. *Br J Urol* 1989;64:594–599.
46. Langer R, Neuman M, Ron-El R, et al: The effect of total abdominal hysterectomy on bladder function in asymptomatic women. *Obstet Gynecol* 1989;74:205–207.
47. Sand PK, Bowen LW, Ostergard DR, et al: Hysterectomy and prior incontinence surgery as risk factors for failed retropubic urethropexy. *J Reprod Med* 1988;33:171–174.
48. Langer R, Ron-El R, Neuman M, et al: The value of simultaneous hysterectomy during Burch colposuspension for urinary stress incontinence. *Obstet Gynecol* 1988;72:866–869.

49. Stanton SL, Cardozo LD: Results of the colposuspension operation for incontinence and prolapse. *Br J Obstet Gynaecol* 1979;86:693–697.
50. Storer EH: Appendix, in Schwartz SI (ed): *Principles of Surgery*, ed 3. New York, McGraw-Hill, 1979, pp 1257–1267.
51. Melcher DH: Appendectomy with abdominal hysterectomy. *Lancet* 1971;1:810–811.
52. Waters EG: Elective appendectomy with abdominal and pelvic surgery. *Obstet Gynecol* 1977;50:511–517.
53. Loeffler F, Stearn R: Abdominal hysterectomy with appendectomy. *Acta Obstet Gynecol Scand* 167;46:435–443.
54. Voitk AJ, Lowry JB: Is incidental appendectomy a safe practice? *Can J Surg* 1988;31:448–451.
55. McGowan L: Incidental appendectomy during vaginal surgery. *Am J Obstet Gynecol* 1966;95:588.
56. Pratt JH, O'Leary JA, Symmonds RE: Combined cholecystectomy and hysterectomy: A study of 95 cases. *Mayo Clin Proc* 1967;42:529–535.
57. Murray JM, Gilstrap LC, Massey FM: Cholecystectomy and abdominal hysterectomy. *JAMA* 1980;244:2305–2306.
58. Hester TR, Baird W, Bostwick J, et al: Abdominoplasty combined with other major surgical procedures: Safe or sorry? *Plast Reconstr Surg* 1989;83:997–1004.
59. Floros C, David PKB: Complications and long-term results following abdominoplasty: A retrospective study. *Br J Plast Surg* 1991;44:190–194.
60. Voss SC, Sharp HC, Scott JR: Abdominoplasty combined with gynecologic surgical procedures. *Obstet Gynecol* 1986;67:181–186.
61. Kovac SR: Vaginal hysterectomy combined with liposuction. *Mo Med* 1989;86:165–168.

Chapter 9

Hysterectomy in the Face of Pelvic Inflammatory Disease

David E. Soper, MD

In the last decade, over 200,000 women from 15 to 44 years of age were hospitalized for pelvic inflammatory disease (PID). Surgery was performed during 42% of hospitalizations for acute PID and in over 90% of hospitalizations for chronic PID. Hysterectomy or other pelvic organ removal was performed in more than one third of patients with acute PID and in more than two thirds with chronic PID.[1] The surgical management of PID with laparotomy is being replaced by an increased emphasis on laparoscopic confirmation of the diagnosis followed by a conservative approach to treatment based primarily on the administration of antibiotics. In addition, endoscopic management of selected cases of severe PID further decreases the necessity for more invasive surgical procedures. Laparotomy and extirpative surgery, including hysterectomy, remain useful in selected cases.

Pathophysiology

Pelvic inflammatory disease is the result of an ascending infection by bacteria that have colonized the endocervix. The most commonly incriminated microorganisms are the sexually transmitted pathogens, *Neisseria gonorrhoeae* and *Chlamydia trachomatis*.[2] Infection of the endocervix with these pathogens results in inflammation (endocervicitis). With ascending spread, these pathogens produce inflammation throughout the upper genital tract (endometritis, salpingitis, and peritonitis). Respiratory pathogens, such as *Haemophilus influenzae, Streptococcus pneumoniae*, and *Streptococcus pyogenes*, are found in approximately 5% of cases.[3] These microorganisms appear able to reach the upper genital tract through canalicular spread (capillary tube action). Retrograde menstruation may play a role in contaminating the fallopian tubes and peritoneum with microorganisms.

A polymicrobial infection with aerobic and anaerobic bacteria has been identified in 30% to 40% of patients with laparoscopically proven acute salpingitis.[3-6] The source of these microorganisms is unclear. Sweet[7] has noted that the isolates obtained from the endometrial cavity are similar to those in the fallopian tube in patients with acute salpingitis. Eschenbach et al[8] reported an association of bacterial vaginosis with a clinical diagnosis of PID. This evidence suggests that ascending infection by these potential pathogens occurs.

Tuboovarian abscess (TOA) formation, the most severe consequence of PID, complicates approximately 15% of PID cases. The pathophysiology is identical to uncomplicated salpingitis except that, presumably through an ovulation site, microorganisms enter the ovarian stroma. This leads to destruction of the ovary and formation of an abscess cavity. Collections of pus can develop between the tube, ovary, uterus, and bowel. These loculations act as abscesses and destroy adjacent pelvic organs. Pyosalpinges are collections of pus within terminally occluded fallopian tubes. The microbiology of TOAs is predominantly anaerobic.[9] The anaerobic infection may be the result of an initial infection by *N. gonorrhoeae* or *C. trachomatis* that causes an alteration in local factors, permitting the development of a polymicrobial superinfection.[10] Alternatively, intrauterine procedures (ie, intrauterine contraceptive device [IUD] insertion, hysterosalpingogram, dilation and suction curettage for therapeutic abortion) may introduce microorganisms from the upper vagina and endocervix into the endometrium and subsequently the fallopian tube.

Actinomyces israelii is a rare cause of severe salpingitis and TOA formation. This microorganism causes an ascending infection of the endometrium, fallopian tubes, ovaries, and peritoneum or infects the pelvic organs from the bowel via appendiceal rupture. Clinical manifestations of this disease are protean. Patients frequently have long-standing abdominal pain and a palpable pelvic mass. Many patients undergo exploratory laparotomy with a preoperative diagnosis of cancer. The most significant predisposing factors that appear are colonization of the cervix and vagina with *Actinomyces* and the use of an IUD. Diagnosis in these areas is usually made at the time of exploratory laparotomy when signs of infection are found, and histologic specimens confirm the presence of *Actinomyces*.[11]

Diagnosis

The most common symptom of patients with PID is lower abdominal pain. This pain is usually bilateral and diffuse throughout the lower abdominal quadrants. Metrorrhagia (intermenstrual spotting) is an important associated symptom. It is evidence of endometritis. Abnormal vaginal discharge and postcoital vaginal bleeding, symptoms associated with endocervicitis, may also be present. Urinary frequency, urgency, and dysuria may be due to an associated urethritis caused by *C. trachomatis* or

N. gonorrhoeae. Nausea and vomiting may occur infrequently, with proctitis symptoms occurring less often. Fever is present in fewer than half of the patients with PID.

The most important clinical sign of acute salpingitis is the presence of a lower genital tract infection (LGTI). A LGTI is heralded by the presence of leukorrhea and/or cervical mucopus. Leukorrhea is defined as the presence of more than one leukocyte per epithelial cell when microscopy (400× magnification, high dry) is performed on a saline preparation of the vaginal secretions. The presence of cervical mucopus also suggests endocervicitis, and cervical mucopus is inevitably present in the patient with salpingitis. Mucopus is present when a Gram's-stained smear of endocervical mucus shows more than 30 leukocytes per oil immersion field. A less specific but more expedient way of determining the presence of mucopus is to remove the external cervical secretions with a large swab and then use a cotton-tipped applicator to sample the endocervical mucus. If the mucus is yellow or green, then mucopus is present and a diagnosis of endocervicitis can be made. Patients without signs of a LGTI, rarely (less than 5% of the time) have salpingitis.

In most cases of PID, a bimanual pelvic examination will reveal bilateral adnexal tenderness. Cervical motion tenderness is a common finding, but the classic "chandelier sign" (the patient lifts her buttocks off the examining table with manual manipulation of the cervix) occurs only in patients with severe clinical disease. Direct and indirect lower abdominal tenderness reflects the amount of pelvic peritonitis. Most PID is associated with a limited amount of abdominal tenderness and rigidity, because peritonitis may be limited to the pelvis and the abdominal wall lacks representation of those muscles that line the pelvic cavity.[12] Patients with severe disease or with TOA formation may have a palpable mass in the adnexa or cul-de-sac. This mass is generally ill defined and represents an agglutination of the pelvic organs with loops of small and large bowel. Fever is present in less than half of patients with PID. Chlamydial salpingitis is more indolent and may not be associated with fever.

Laboratory tests that are helpful in the diagnosis of PID include a white blood cell count and either a C-reactive protein (CRP) level or erythrocyte sedimentation rate (ESR). Leukocytosis is present in almost 60% of patients with acute salpingitis. A CRP level greater than 2 mg/dL has a strong correlation with laparoscopically confirmed salpingitis in patients with the clinical diagnosis of PID. An ESR greater than 15 mm/h is present in 75% of patients with acute salpingitis.

The accuracy of the diagnosis of PID is based on the individual patient's composite clinical criteria. Patients with the triad of lower abdominal pain, bilateral adnexal tenderness, and leukorrhea have a 61% chance of having laparoscopically confirmed acute salpingitis. Patients with these classical symptoms and signs of PID plus the presence of fever and leukocytosis have a very high probability of having laparoscopically confirmable disease.[13]

Related Conditions

Chronic Pelvic Inflammatory Disease

The term "chronic PID" suggests long-term chronic infection and is therefore a misnomer. In reality, chronic PID is the sequelae of pelvic adhesions and distorted tubal anatomy, such as hydrosalpinx formation, following an episode(s) of acute PID. Severe PID with TOA formation is actually a complication of acute PID and represents a continuum within that disease. Two significant exceptions to this statement occur with respect to PID caused by *A. israelii* and *Mycobacterium tuberculosis*. Infection with these slow-growing microorganisms can take months to become clinically recognizable.

Atypical or "Silent" Salpingitis

More than half of women with tubal factor infertility have no history of PID. Antibodies to *C. trachomatis* are often present in asymptomatic women with either ectopic pregnancy or distal tubal occlusion. Moreover, morphologic changes of the fallopian tube mucosa and physiologic alterations of its ciliated epithelium are similar in patients with tubal factor infertility with and without a history of PID.[14] Endometrial infection with *C. trachomatis* has been documented in asymptomatic women with antichlamydial antibodies.[15] These data suggest that patients develop salpingitis without the typical clinical signs of pelvic infection. In some cases, pelvic pain is absent and symptoms such as metrorrhagia or abnormal vaginal discharge, or urinary tract symptoms, may represent the clinical manifestations of PID. It would not be uncommon to detect "chronic PID" (pelvic adhesions and hydrosalpinx formation) in these women.

Fitz-Hugh-Curtis Syndrome

Fitz-Hugh-Curtis syndrome is characterized by violin string adhesions between the liver and the diaphragm in women with gross pathologic evidence of prior tubal infection. Acute salpingitis leads to acute perihepatitis and results in the formation of perihepatic adhesions. Both *N. gonorrhoeae* and *C. trachomatis* have been isolated from the liver capsule in patients with perihepatitis. Acute perihepatitis can mimic the clinical presentation of acute cholecystitis. Normal liver function tests in patients with perihepatitis helps distinguish between the two. In addition, patients with perihepatitis have signs of PID, including leukorrhea. Patients with Fitz-Hugh-Curtis syndrome respond to the same antibiotic regimens as are used to treat PID. The severity of their liver adhesions correlates with the severity of their pelvic adhesions, suggesting that both processes are progressive. Occasionally, the chronic right upper quadrant pain associated with Fitz-Hugh-Curtis syndrome will be so disabling as to suggest the need for laparoscopic lysis of adhesions.

Laparoscopy

The gold standard for the diagnosis of PID involves laparoscopic confirmation of tubal inflammation. Minimum findings necessary for the visual confirmation of salpingitis are (1) hyperemia of the tubal surface, (2) edema of the tubal wall, and (3) a sticky exudate on the tubal surface and from the fimbriated ends when patent.[13]

Routine use of diagnostic laparoscopy to confirm the presence of acute salpingitis allows determination of the extent of the disease and is helpful in following its clinical course. Patients with severe salpingitis can be expected to require a longer course of antibiotic therapy before a clinical response is observed.[6] Laparoscopy allows the clinician to obtain reliable cultures. These cultures, although not immediately helpful in choosing an antibiotic regimen, are helpful if the patient fails to respond to initial antibiotic treatment. In those cases in which sensitive microorganisms are present, more prolonged treatment or surgical intervention is needed. In those cases in which a resistant microorganism is present, a change in antibiotic regimen is warranted. Laparoscopy is also helpful as a predictor of reproductive potential. Patients with mild disease have a better prognosis with regard to their future fertility than do patients with severe disease. In addition, there may be some advantage in using laparoscopy for the removal of free pus from the pelvis, for aspiration of pyosalpinges, and for lysis of adhesions. Future study is needed of an aggressive laparoscopic approach and its impact on the preservation of reproductive function.

A dichotomy exists in determining candidates for diagnostic laparoscopy. The patient with significant symptoms of PID is considered to be a plausible candidate for surgery. In contrast, the mildly ill patient, who may not otherwise receive therapy for salpingitis, probably has the most to gain from early diagnosis. Not all medical centers are able to offer routine laparoscopy for the diagnosis of PID. Moreover, not all investigators believe that routine laparoscopic diagnosis is necessary for the management of PID. It appears clear, however, that there are several clinical situations that warrant the use of diagnostic laparoscopy. First, in those cases in which the diagnosis is in question, especially if ectopic pregnancy is a possibility, laparoscopy should be performed. In addition, persistent symptoms in women treated as outpatients for PID are an indication of the need for diagnostic laparoscopy. Patients who fail to respond to outpatient antibiotic therapy rarely have laparoscopically confirmed acute salpingitis. In fact, many have an alternative, yet treatable, disease such as endometriosis. Another scenario that should prompt diagnostic laparoscopy includes patients with a past history of multiple episodes of PID, usually treated on an outpatient basis, who have signs and symptoms suggestive of recurrent disease. These patients benefit from diagnostic laparoscopy to confirm the diagnosis, assess the microbial etiology, determine the extent of disease, and rule out an alternative or coexisting diagnosis such as endometriosis.

Once the diagnosis of acute salpingitis has been visually confirmed, grading of the severity of the disease should be undertaken. The grading system is based primarily on the mobility and patency of the fallopian tubes.[13] Mild salpingitis is associated with freely mobile, patent fallopian tubes that meet the minimum criteria for the diagnosis of salpingitis. Moderate disease is associated with more pronounced inflammation. Patchy fibrin deposits may be seen on the serosal surfaces, tubes are not freely mobile, the fimbria may be adherent and associated with some paraphimosis, and adhesions are loose and moist. Severe disease is associated with intensely congested peritoneal surfaces. Pelvic organs adhere to each other, pyosalpinx or tuboovarian complex formation may have occurred, and omental adhesions may be present. Each adnexa should be graded independently, with the overall grade assigned being equal to the most severe findings.

The definition of a TOA is somewhat problematic. In patients not undergoing diagnostic laparoscopy, a palpable mass associated with the clinical signs and symptoms of PID is considered a TOA. Laparoscopic findings of severe disease may include a freely mobile, but occluded and distended, fallopian tube. This represents a tubal abscess that may or may not involve adjacent pelvic organs. More common findings associated with TOA include loculations of purulent fluid between the adnexa and the uterus, usually with some involvement of the bowel. Both tubal abscesses and ovarian abscesses may be involved in these complexes.

The laparoscopic grade of disease may be out of proportion to the clinical severity of disease. This is due to cases in which acute infection is superimposed on preexisting pelvic adhesive disease. These patients will have a more advanced grade of disease when, in fact, the amount of purulent exudate, side-to-side agglutination, and tubal edema and erythema may be less than with an initial mild grade of gonococcal salpingitis.

Treatment

Centers for Disease Control guidelines for the treatment of PID reflect the concern that a significant number of cases will be associated with polymicrobial infection. Recommended regimens provide empiric coverage of likely etiologic pathogens while maintaining an emphasis on coverage of both *N. gonorrhoeae* and *C. trachomatis*. Table 9.1 lists appropriate antibiotic regimens.[16]

The outpatient management of PID utilizes a single dose of a β-lactam antibiotic such as ceftriaxone, followed by 10 to 14 days of oral doxycycline. This regimen has excellent activity against both *N. gonorrhoeae* and *C. trachomatis*. However, it provides little in the way of coverage for a significant anaerobic soft tissue infection. For this reason, patients suspected of having anaerobic infections, such as those associated with TOA formation or IUD use, should be hospitalized for more broad-spectrum antibiotic therapy. All patients treated as outpatients should return for

Table 9.1 1989 Centers for Disease Control Treatment Guidelines for PID

Inpatient Treatment

Regimen A
  Cefoxitin 2 g IV very 6 h, *or* cefotetan[a] 2 g IV every 12 h
  PLUS
  Doxycycline 100 mg every 12 hours orally or IV
Regimen B
  Clindamycin 900 mg IV every 8 h
  PLUS
  Gentamicin loading dose IV or IM (2 mg/kg) followed by a maintenance dose (1.5 mg/kg) every 8 h
One of the above regimens is given for at least 48 h after the patient clinically improves.
After discharge from the hospital, continuation of:
  Doxycycline 100 mg orally two times daily to total 10–14 d (clindamycin 450 mg orally five times daily for 10–14 d may be considered as an alternative)

Outpatient Treatment

Cefoxitin 2 g IM plus probenecid, 1 g orally concurrently *or* ceftriaxone 250 mg IM, or equivalent cephalosporin
PLUS
Doxycycline 100 mg orally two times daily for 10–14 d
or
Tetracycline 500 mg orally four times daily for 10–14 d
Alternative for patients not tolerating doxycycline is erythromycin, 500 mg orally four times daily for 10–14 d

From Centers for Disease Control: 1989 sexually transmitted diseases treatment guidelines. *MMWR* 1989;38:31.

[a] Other cephalosporins such as ceftizoxime, cefotaxime, and ceftriaxone, which provide adequate gonococcal, other facultative gram-negative aerobic, and anaerobic coverage, may be utilized in appropriate doses.

---

repeat evaluation (symptoms, bimanual pelvic examination, repeat white blood cell count, and CRP level) within 72 hours. If no clinical response is noted, hospital admission and diagnostic laparoscopy should be considered.

Ideally, all patients with the clinical diagnosis of PID should be admitted for parenteral antibiotic therapy. This approach ensures patient compliance and allows broad-spectrum antibiotic coverage until the patient has had a clinical response. However, no data exist to suggest that inpatient therapy is superior to ambulatory therapy. Hospitalization has a dramatic impact on the cost of treatment for PID and, therefore, alternative approaches based primarily on the severity of clinical disease have been adopted. Some patients may benefit from hospitalization. Patients with severe clinical disease and/or those who are unable to tolerate oral antibiotic therapy should be admitted for treatment. In addition, adolescents, because they poorly comply with an outpatient oral antibiotic regimen, should be admitted, if possible, for observation and parenteral therapy. Recommended inpatient antibiotic regimens provide broad-spectrum coverage for infection by the sexually transmitted pathogens and for mixed infections of aerobic and anaerobic microorganisms. The combination of cefoxitin and doxycycline provides excellent activity against *N. gonorrhoeae* and *C. trachomatis* in addition to anaerobic microorganisms. Cefoxitin also is effective against mixed infections caused by aerobic gram-negative bacteria and the penicillinase-producing *Bac-*

teroides species. The combination of clindamycin and gentamicin provides adequate coverage of *N. gonorrhoeae* and *C. trachomatis* and excellent coverage of the mixed aerobic and anaerobic bacteria. Clindamycin appears to be especially helpful in the treatment of pelvic abscesses. This antibiotic concentrates within leukocytes and therefore is particularly effective in abscess cavities because the leukocytes act as vehicles to transport the antibiotic into the site of infection.

For hospitalized patients, parenteral antibiotic therapy should be continued until a therapeutic response is obtained. Criteria for switching to oral antibiotic treatment and for discharge from the hospital should include lysis of fever (temperature less than 99.5°F for 24 hours), normalization of the white blood cell count, total disappearance of abdominal rebound tenderness, and marked amelioration of pelvic organ tenderness. A pelvic examination prior to the patient's discharge is important. Not only can significant pelvic tenderness remain after the disappearance of abdominal tenderness, but previously undetected pelvic masses may also be found.

Treatment of PID involves more than just antibiotic therapy. Sexual partners of patients treated for PID should be evaluated for sexually transmitted diseases. Screening these individuals may suggest the pathogenesis of PID in the culture-negative patient as well as identify a reservoir for reinfection. Approximately one third of male sexual contacts of patients with gonococcal PID will test positive for the gonococcus, and many will be asymptomatic. Moreover, even sexual contacts of patients with nongonococcal PID will have a 15% incidence of culture-proven *N. gonorrhoeae* infection.[17] In addition, chlamydia infection is present in 35% of the sexual partners of women with PID.[18] Sexual contacts should be treated with ceftriaxone and doxycycline for uncomplicated LGTIs caused by *N. gonorrhoeae* or *C. trachomatis*.

Surgical Management

The initial surgical approach to the management of PID involves the use of diagnostic laparoscopy to confirm the diagnosis and grade of the disease. These principles have been discussed. There also may be some benefit in the use of operative endoscopy at the time of initial laparoscopy to lyse adhesions, aspirate pyosalpinges, dissect and drain loculations of pus, and irrigate the pelvic and abdominal cavity. These manipulations are safe, but the surgeon must be careful to avoid harming the patient. Tissues in an acute phase of inflammation are more friable, and harsh probing has the potential for laceration and/or perforation. Extirpation of pelvic organs should be reserved for cases that have failed to respond to an initial course of antibiotic therapy.

Although laparotomy is not usually required in managing PID, three clinical situations are associated with its use: (1) generalized peritonitis associated with signs of sepsis caused by a ruptured TOA; (2) exploratory laparotomy for an alternative preoperative diagnosis, with PID being discovered; and (3) severe PID with TOA formation that is refractory to medical therapy.[19] Determination of the extent of disease and the patient's desire for future fertility should define the limits of extirpative surgery.

When laparotomy is undertaken, a great deal of surgical judgment must be used to determine the extent of extirpative surgery. In patients who desire future fertility, a conservative approach is recommended. This may involve unilateral adnexectomy if the disease is predominantly one sided. In cases of severe bilateral disease, partial bilateral adnexectomy without hysterectomy may be performed. Patients without adnexa are still able to conceive with the help of in vitro fertilization programs. Extensive irrigation of the pelvic cavity is warranted, with drainage of collections of purulent material. In patients who have finished childbearing, total abdominal hysterectomy and bilateral salpingo-oophorectomy should be performed. In cases associated with diffuse severe pelvic disease, with or without associated systemic signs of sepsis, total abdominal hysterectomy and bilateral salpingo-oophorectomy may be necessary regardless of the patient's wishes.

The following facts should be considered in the management of a patient taken to the operating room with an acute abdomen, with or without signs of a small bowel obstruction, in whom salpingitis is discovered. It is important to know the age and reproductive desires of the patient. If these are unknown, the surgeon should choose a conservative surgical approach. Remember that over 90% of patients with PID will respond to antibiotic treatment alone, so initial extirpative surgery is probably ill advised. Remember also that the pelvic organs may actually look worse than the clinical presentation of the patient would suggest. This is especially true of chlamydia-associated salpingitis. Seventy percent of patients with TOAs will respond to antibiotic therapy alone; therefore, a conservative surgical approach utilizing drainage and irrigation without extirpation of the pelvic organs appears to be the most judicious approach when the reproductive desires of the patient are unknown.

An additional indication for surgical intervention by laparotomy occurs when the patient with a TOA has failed to respond to appropriate antibiotic therapy. Initial management of the patient with a TOA should include antibiotic therapy utilizing an agent with an excellent antianaerobic spectrum, such as clindamycin or metronidazole. The patient should be given 72 to 96 hours to respond to therapy, with pain, abdominal tenderness, white blood cell count, and CRP level decreasing. Documentation and assessment of the size of the abscess should be undertaken with pelvic ultrasound or computerized tomography. If the patient's clinical status deteriorates or if, after 72 to 96 hours of antibiotic treatment, a response to therapy has not been appreciated, surgical exploration is advisable. The operation performed should take into consideration the patient's desire for fertility and hormone production and the extent of the disease.

In some cases, a cul-de-sac abscess will complicate PID, and the patients affected may well be refractory to antibiotic therapy and require surgical intervention. If significant dissection along the rectovaginal septum has taken place, a colpotomy incision may be the least morbid approach to the drainage of the pelvic abscess. Following incision and drainage of the abscess, a large Malecot drain should be placed in the abscess cavity to allow continued drainage. This drain may be removed when the patient has responded to treatment and all drainage has ceased.

In selected cases, percutaneous drainage under guidance from ultrasound or computerized tomography can be useful. Unilocular abscesses are the type of collections most successfully drained in this manner. Since the majority of TOAs are multilocular and are intimately involved with both the large and small bowel, this approach has only limited utility in managing TOAs.

Hysterectomy

When exploratory surgery becomes necessary, the abdomen should be opened through a midline incision. Tuboovarian abscesses are usually bilateral and, when total abdominal hysterectomy and bilateral salpingo-oophorectomy are indicated, adequate exposure is imperative. Landmarks of normal pelvic architecture are commonly obliterated, and the operation challenges even the superior surgeon's skill. Commonly, the small and large bowel are agglutinated to the pelvic structures and the tubes and ovaries are involved in inflammatory masses associated with adhesions and loculation of pus.

The first order of business, after lysing bowel adhesions and draining any accumulated pus, is to start with the pelvic structures that can be identified. This usually is one or both of the round ligaments, which can be elevated with a clamp, ligated, and divided. This is the easiest way to begin such a pelvic dissection.[20] Entrance into the retroperitoneum occurs after dissection of the pelvic side wall peritoneum attached to the round ligaments. Exploitation of these spaces (the paravesical and pararectal spaces) allows for the safe identification of the infundibulopelvic ligament and pelvic ureter. The ovarian vasculature can then be carefully freed from any attachments to an inflammatory mass or bowel, ligated, and divided. Continued dissection of the peritoneum above the pelvic ureter and toward the uterus will mobilize the adnexa. Adnexectomy can then be accomplished if conservative surgical therapy is deemed appropriate.

The peritoneum is frequently edematous, making identification of the bladder difficult. Meticulous sharp dissection should be used to reflect the bladder from the cervix and upper vagina. Skeletonization of the uterine vasculature can then be accomplished, allowing these vessels to be clamped, divided, and ligated. The hysterectomy can then be completed without difficulty in most cases. However, brawny induration associated with ligneous pelvic cellulitis may make dissection of the cardinal ligaments difficult. These findings are particularly striking in actinomycotic pelvic infection. Mature surgical judgment concerning the advisability of a subtotal hysterectomy should be exercised.[21]

Irrigation of the abdominal and pelvic cavities should be performed, and careful exploration of the upper abdomen and bowel should ensure that all interloop abscesses and free pus have been drained. Antibiotics added to the irrigant offer no advantage over irrigation with normal saline alone.

Drainage of the operative site should be established following hysterectomy. A Malecot drain may be placed through an open vaginal cuff, allowing dependent drainage of the pelvis. Alternatively, the vaginal cuff may be closed and a Jackson-Pratt suction drain may be placed overlying the operative site.

Closure of the abdominal incision requires close attention. Patients undergoing abdominal hysterectomy with salpingo-oophorectomy for pelvic abscess are at increased risk for wound dehiscence. Nasogastric suction should be considered to decrease postoperative bowel distention. These patients should undergo mass closure of the fascia utilizing nonabsorbable monofilament suture material. In addition, the subcutaneous tissue and skin should initially be packed open and either undergo delayed primary closure or be allowed to heal by secondary intention.[22] This allows the clinician to assess the patient's response to continued antibiotic therapy in the postoperative period without having to worry about a wound infection as the source of persistent fever if this occurs.

Summary

Pelvic inflammatory diseases continues to be a common finding in young women with lower abdominal pain. Typical emergency room PID, with classic symptoms of pain, fever, and a history of high-risk sexual behavior, is easily diagnosed with a high degree of specificity. However, the majority of patients with PID have atypical symptoms and may actually be incorrectly diagnosed and not treated. Careful attention to the physical signs of pelvic infection and the evaluation of the vaginal secretions for leukocytes improves diagnostic accuracy. Liberal use of diagnostic laparoscopy to confirm the possibility of acute salpingitis is recommended in young women who have much to lose from a case of untreated salpingitis. Outpatient treatment with a β-lactam antibiotic, followed by a course of doxycycline, adequately treats patients with *N. gonorrhoeae* and *C. trachomatis* infections. However, patients with suspected anaerobic upper genital tract infection, such as those associated with TOA or IUD use, should be admitted for parenteral antibiotic therapy and observation. Laparotomy and extirpative surgery should be reserved for seriously ill patients with generalized peritonitis associated with rupture of a TOA, for patients who do not respond to antibiotic therapy, and for patients with chronic pelvic pain caused by pelvic adhesions (chronic PID). Sound judgment regarding the extent of extirpative surgery, taking into consideration the wishes of the patient with respect to future fertility and hormone production, will lead to an acceptable outcome. Unfortunately, hysterectomy is unavoidable in many clinical situations. Exploitation of the retroperitoneal spaces allows for the safe completion of this operation. Drainage of the operative site is an important part of the surgical approach to the patient with persistent PID. Judicious managment of the abdominal wound can decrease the risk of postoperative wound infection and disruption associated with these cases.

References

1. Rolfs RT, Galaid EI, Zaidi AA: Pelvic inflammatory disease: Trends in hospitalizations and office visits, 1979–1988. *Am J Obstet Gynecol* 1992;166:938–990.
2. Mardh PA: An overview of infectious agents of salpingitis, their biology, and recent advances in methods of detection. *Am J Obstet Gynecol* 1980;138: 933–951.
3. Burnham RC, Binns B, Guijon F, et al: Etiology and outcome of acute pelvic inflammatory disease. *J Infect Dis* 1988;158:510–517.
4. Soper DE, Brockwell NJ, Dalton HP: Pathogenesis of urban emergency room PID: Treatment with ofloxacin. Read at the annual meeting of the Infectious Disease Society for Obstetrics/Gynecology, Seattle, Oct, 1990.
5. Sweet RL, Draper DL, Hadley WK: Etiology of acute salpingitis: Influence of episode number and duration of symptoms. *Obstet Gynecol* 1981;58:62–68.
6. Wasserheit JN, Bell TA, Kiviat NB, et al: Microbial causes of proven pelvic inflammatory disease and efficacy of clindamycin and tobramycin. *Ann Intern Med* 1986;104:187–193.
7. Sweet RL: Pelvic inflammatory disease, in Sweet RL, Gibbs RS (eds): *Infectious Diseases of the Female Genital Tract*, ed 2. Baltimore, Williams & Wilkins, 1990.
8. Eschenbach DA, Hillier S, Critchlow C, et al: Diagnosis and clinical manifestations of bacterial vaginosis. *Am J Obstet Gynecol* 1988;158:819–828.
9. Landers DV, Sweet RL: Current trends in the diagnosis and treatment of tubo-ovarian abscess. *Am J Obstet Gynecol* 1985;151:1098–1110.
10. Monif GRG: Significance of polymicrobial bacterial superinfection in the therapy of gonococcal endometritis-salpingitis-peritonitis. *Obstet Gynecol* 1980; 55:154S–161S.
11. Schmidt WA, Bedrossian CWM, Ali V, et al: Actinomycosis and intrauterine contraceptive devices: The clinicopathologic entity. *Diagn Gynecol Obstet* 1980;2:165–177.
12. Cope Z: Appendicitis, in *The Early Diagnosis of the Acute Abdomen*. New York, Oxford University Press, 1972.

13. Westrom L, Mardh P-A: Salpingitis, in Holmes KK, Mardh P-A, Sparling PF, et al (eds): *Sexually Transmitted Diseases*. New York, McGraw-Hill, 1984.
14. Patton DL, Moore DE, Spadoni LR, et al: A comparison of the fallopian tube's response to overt and silent salpingitis. *Obstet Gynecol* 1989;73:622–630.
15. Cleary RE, Jones RB: Recovery of *Chlamydia trachomatis* from the endometrium in infertile women with serum antichylamydial antibodies. *Fertil Steril* 1985;44:233–235.
16. Centers for Disease Control: 1989 sexually transmitted disease treatment guidelines. *MMWR* 1989;38:1–43.
17. Gilstrap LC, Herbert WNP, Cunningham FG, et al: Gonorrhea screening in male consorts of women with pelvic infection. *JAMA* 1977;238:965–966.
18. Moss TR, Hawkswell J: Evidence of infection with *Chlamydia trachomatis* in patients with pelvic inflammatory disease: Value of partner investigation. *Fertil Steril* 1986;45:429–430.
19. Soper DE: Surgical considerations in the diagnosis and treatment of pelvic inflammatory disease. *Surg Clin North Am* 1991;71:947–962.
20. Benigno BB: Medical and surgical management of the pelvic abscess. *Clin Obstet Gynecol* 1981;24:1187–1197.
21. Mattingly RF, Thompson JD: Pelvic inflammatory disease, in Mattingly RF, Thompson JD (eds): *TeLinde's Operative Gynecology*, ed 6. Philadelphia, JB Lippincott, 1985.
22. Brown SE, Allen HH, Robins RN: The use of delayed primary wound closure in preventing wound infections. *Am J Obstet Gynecol* 1977;127:713–717.

Chapter 10

Postoperative Care

W. Glenn Hurt, MD

The postoperative care of a patient who has undergone a hysterectomy depends more on the patient's general medical condition, operative findings, and ancillary procedures than it does on the route, vaginal or abdominal, through which the uterus is removed. Although there are standard procedures for the postoperative care of all hysterectomy patients, each patient's postoperative orders must be designed to meet her own personal needs.

As soon as the surgical procedure is completed, the surgeon has four immediate responsibilities: (1) enter a postoperative note into the medical record; (2) enter postoperative orders into the medical record; (3) dictate the operative procedure; and (4) talk with the patient's family about her surgery and her overall condition. Examples of a postoperative note and basic postoperative orders are shown in Tables 10.1 and 10.2, although the orders are subject to modifications for each patient.

There are reports in the surgical literature of women who have had hysterectomies performed on an outpatient basis. If a woman is to have a hysterectomy on an outpatient basis, it is assumed that she is in excellent physical condition, that the surgical procedure is not complicated, and that she has a capable person to remain with her during the immediate postoperative period. A telephone and a means of transportation to a hospital also should be available.

This chapter is concerned with the routine postoperative care of hospitalized patients who have a vaginal or abdominal hysterectomy for a benign gynecologic disorder.

Recovery Room Care

Recovery room personnel are responsible for monitoring vital functions and providing respiratory support as the patient emerges from anesthesia and until the respiratory and cardiovascular systems are stable. They accomplish this by maintaining an airway and observing respiratory functions, blood pressure, electrocardiogram, hematologic parameters, and

Table 10.1 Outline Format for a Standard Postoperative Note

1. Preoperative diagnosis
2. Intraoperative findings
3. Postoperative diagnosis
4. Surgeon's name
5. Anesthesia (eg, general, regional)
6. Anesthesiologist's name
7. Estimated blood loss; blood administered
8. Fluids administered
9. Packs, drains, etc
10. Sheet, sponge, needle, and instrument count
11. Complications
12. Condition in recovery room
13. Signature of physician entering operative note

urinary output. If they provide adequate pain control, it will help prevent agitation and promote the return of normal physiologic processes.[1,2]

In the immediate postoperative period, common respiratory complications include airway obstruction, hypoxemia, and hyperventilation with carbon dioxide retention. Common circulatory complications include bleeding, hypotension, hypertension, and development of a cardiac arrhythmia. Oliguria (urinary output of less than 30 mL/h in the absence of urinary tract obstruction) is usually due to inadequate intravascular volume or to urinary retention. Failure to increase the urinary output by the intravenous administration of a fluid load may indicate continued intravascular contraction, occult bleeding, or impaired cardiac or renal function.[3]

Table 10.2 Outline Format for Postoperative Orders

1. Postoperative diagnosis
2. Surgical procedures performed
3. Drug allergies
4. Condition: stable, other (specify)
5. Vital signs: each 15 min until stable, then hourly × 4, then every 4 h
6. Notify physician if: blood pressure <90/60 or >160/100; pulse <60 or >120; temperature >100 °F orally
7. Activity: bed rest, progressive ambulation, other (specify)
8. Diet': NPO, sips of clear liquids after nausea; other (specify)
9. Intravenous therapy: dextrose 5% with Ringer's lactate at 125 mL/h; other (specify)
10. Turn, cough, and deep breath every 2 h; encourage inspirometer use
11. Drains: bladder, other (specify)
12. Record fluid intake and output
13. Notify physician if urinary output <30 mL/h
14. Catheterize bladder each 6 h, or sooner if bladder is full and patient unable to void
15. Medictions (specify drug, dosage, route, and frequency of administration)
16. Hematocrit on postoperative days 1 and 3
17. Special orders for the individual patient
18. Signature and pager number of physician entering postoperative orders

Components of Postoperative Care
Hemogram and Transfusions

A patient whose hysterectomy is likely to require a transfusion should be considered a candidate for autologous blood donation.[4] She is a candidate for preoperative donation if her hemoglobin is greater than 11 g/dL (hematocrit greater than 33%) and if there will be at least 3 days between her last blood donation and the day of surgery. All patients undergoing hysterectomy should have a preoperative hemoglobin and/or hematocrit determination. In uncomplicated cases, the hemoglobin and/or hematocrit determination should be performed following the last autologous blood donation and within 10 days of the operation. Preoperative oral iron therapy (ferrous sulfate, ferrous fumarate, or ferrous gluconate) is recommended to correct an iron-deficiency anemia or to help the patient compensate for iron loss as a result of autologous blood donation.

If there has been significant bleeding or a need for a preoperative blood transfusion, a hemoglobin and/or hematocrit determination should be repeated just prior to the surgical procedure. Such a determination should be repeated during surgery and in the recovery room, as dictated by the amount of operative blood loss or by changes in the patient's blood pressure and pulse. After recovery, the patient should have at least one postoperative hemoglobin and/or hematocrit determination for documentation of its adequacy. Hemoglobin and/or hematocrit determinations performed within the first 24 hours of major surgical procedures are not as predictive of true values as those performed at least 72 hours following surgery. The patient should have stable hemoglobin and/or hematocrit values, evidence of satisfactory physiologic parameters when erect and ambulating, and no excessive bleeding at the time of discharge from the hospital.

Patients with chronic anemias whose hemoglobin values are 6 to 8 g/dL usually undergo anesthesia and surgery uneventfully. Moderate anemias do not affect some coexisting diseases (eg, coronary artery disease), but an adequate intravascular volume is far more important than red cell mass in providing tissue oxygenation.[5]

I administer autologous blood to patients whose hemoglobin is less than 9 g/dL and nonautologous blood to patients whose hemoglobin is less than 7 g/dL and whose blood pressure and pulse indicate the need for blood. I am aware that there are those who are more liberal in administering autologous blood, but I believe that we should observe some caution in its use. Clerical and/or technical errors may cause a patient to have an adverse reaction to a transfusion; there are changes that might occur as a result of blood preservation and storage that could also cause such reactions. Those administering blood or blood products must be aware of the possibility of transfusion reactions (allergic, febrile, hemolytic) and of the possibility of circulatory collapse.

Fluids and Electrolytes

A record of fluid intake and output (including urinary and gastrointestinal losses) should be kept from the time the patient leaves the operating room until intravenous fluid therapy is discontinued and she is tolerating an oral diet. The afebrile hysterectomy patient will remain in fluid balance if she received 2,500 mL of fluid during the first 24 hours and has no unusual gastrointestinal or insensible fluid losses. When the renal function is normal, this fluid is best administered as a 5% dextrose and lactated Ringer's solution. The daily requirements of fluids and electrolytes (sodium, 150 mEq, and potassium, 40 mEq, each 24 hours) must be supplemented to make up for excessive gastrointestinal, urinary, or third-space losses. In complicated cases (ie, ileus, diarrhea, sepsis, acute renal failure), frequent serum electrolyte determinations and daily weights should be used to guide fluid and electrolyte therapy. Fluid therapy is discontinued when oral intake is adequate in amount and substance.[6]

Pain Control

Postoperative pain often causes patients to be restless and to limit their respiratory effort and their ambulation. Adequate pain control is important for the patient's physical comfort and also to diminish the risk of pulmonary and cardiovascular complications. Unfortunately, the majority of patients who have major surgery do not have adequate postoperative pain control.[7]

Immediate postoperative pain relief is usually provided by administering one of the opiates (morphine, meperidine, hydromorphone, oxycodone, codeine, etc). The drug, the dose, and the frequency of administration may have to be altered to provide adequate pain control. Initially, it is best to administer a pain control drug on a regular schedule to prevent fluctuations in drug levels that might result in unsatisfactory analgesia. The popular alternative is patient-controlled analgesia, which allows the patient to provide small, self-administered intravenous boluses of a drug for pain control. The epidural administration of narcotics can be used to provide postoperative analgesia, but the patient must be monitored closely for respiratory depression if she also requires parenteral narcotics for the relief of pain.[1]

When the patient tolerates liquids, she may be given an oral form of one of the opiates or one of the nonsteroidal antiinflammatory drugs (diflunisal, ibuprofen, naproxen, etc). The latter, however, should be used with caution in patients who are taking anticoagulants or those who have bleeding problems.[1,8]

Bladder Drainage

Postoperative urinary retention may be caused by surgical trauma to the bladder and pelvic nerves, ancillary procedures for the correction of urinary incontinence, and the perioperative administration of parasympatholytic agents and narcotics. There is little difference in the incidence of postoperative urinary retention following the administration of either general or regional anesthesia.

In the hysterectomy patient, continuous bladder drainage is performed too often as a matter of convenience rather than of necessity. Patients who have an uncomplicated hysterectomy for a benign condition and who do not have a concomitant continence procedure can usually be managed with intermittent straight catheterization until they are able to void efficiently. If the patient has been taught self-catheterization, she may prefer to empty her bladder in this manner to maintain comfort and a low urinary residual.

The majority of hysterectomy patients still leave the operating room with an indwelling urinary catheter. I use a transurethral balloon Foley catheter if the anticipated period of postoperative catherization is estimated to be less than 48 to 72 hours. I use a suprapubic bladder catheter if the patient is to be discharged with the catheter in place or if the anticipated period of postoperative catheterization is likely to be greater than 48 to 72 hours. Suprapubic bladder catheters are more comfortable and are more easily managed by patients than are transurethral catheters. In addition, suprapubic bladder catheters are associated with less postoperative infectious morbidity than are transurethral bladder catheters. When voiding trials are undertaken, the patient is instructed to obstruct the outlet of the suprapubic catheter, allow urine to collect in her bladder, and void when she feels the urge to urinate. She then determines the postvoid urinary residual by opening the suprapubic catheter's drainage system and allowing the bladder to drain into an empty urine collection bag. The urinary residual is measured, the collection bag emptied, and the voiding procedure is repeated. The suprapubic catheter is removed when the patient voids at least 200 mL and the postvoid residual is consistently less than 90 mL. This method of bladder management is preferred to that of removing a transurethral balloon catheter, undertaking voiding trials, and then performing repeated transurethral catheterizations in order to determine the postvoid urinary residual. The latter is uncomfortable for the patient and has a high risk of causing urinary tract infections.

My experience is that, when postoperative urinary retention is due to surgical trauma or ancillary continence or prolapse procedures, efficient bladder function usually returns at about the same time as efficient bowel function. Until bladder function occurs, it is important to protect the patient from overdistention of the bladder. One episode of overdistention may delay the return of normal bladder function, damage the urothelium, and contribute to the development of a postoperative urinary tract infection. It is important, therefore, that overdistention of the bladder be prevented, even if it means short-term bladder catheterization.

Bethanechol is of little value in treating postoperative urinary retention. Patients who are unable to void because of periurethral skeletal muscle spasm or anxiety may be helped by the judicious use of diazepam. Prazosin also may be used to reduce urethral resistance.

Reinstitution of Medications

Patients with valvular heart disease who received antibiotic prophylaxis to prevent bacterial endocarditis may need a second dose of antibiotics 8 hours following their surgical procedure. Patients who receive preoperative antibiotic prophylaxis solely to reduce the incidence of postoperative infectious complications do not need additional therapy.[2,9] Patients who received preoperative and/or intraoperative antibiotics for treatment of ongoing infections may need to have their antibiotic therapy continued postoperatively.

Surgeons who choose to administer low-dose heparin as prophylaxis for the prevention of thrombophlebitis and thromboembolic disease should give the first dose (5,000 units, subcutaneously) 2 hours before surgery and that dose should be repeated, subcutaneously, every 12 hours until the patient is fully ambulatory.[2]

Patients who were recently but are not currently on adrenocortical steroids should receive supplemental hydrocortisone 300 mg (100 mg intravenously [IV] or intramuscularly [IM] on call to the operating room and each 8 hours postoperatively) on the day of surgery, 50 mg IV or IM every 8 hours for three doses, and finally 25 mg IV or IM every 8 hours before the medication is discontinued. Patients with postoperative complications (fever, hypotension, etc.) may require an increase in cortisol dosage and a longer tapering period. Patients who are on adrenocorticoid therapy and those with adrenal insufficiency should have their cortisol dosage reduced gradually until they are back to their maintenance level.[2]

A patient's necessary daily medications should be reinstituted as soon as possible in the postoperative period. Parenteral forms of essential medications should be ordered when it is impractical for the patient to take them by mouth. It is important for physicians to be aware of drug interactions and be knowledgeable regarding drugs' adverse reactions. Abrupt discontinuance of propranolol, clonidine, methyldopa, reserpine, and saralasin must be avoided to prevent potential rebound phenomena.[10]

Diabetes may involve the cardiovascular, renal, and nervous systems. The disease also adversely affects wound healing, predisposes the patient to infection, and increases the risk of postoperative venous thromboembolism. Uncontrolled diabetes (hyperglycemia) can lead to electrolyte disturbances, osmotic diuresis, and ketoacidosis. The postoperative blood glucose levels of diabetics should be maintained between 150 and 200 mg/dL.[2]

Diabetics who were well controlled on insulin prior to surgery should receive intravenous fluids containing glucose and one half of their normal insulin dose as regular insulin on the morning of surgery. They should be operated on as promptly as possible. Glucose should be administered intraoperatively as indicated by blood glucose determinations. Postoperative blood glucose determinations should be made every 4 to 6 hours, and regular insulin should be administered subcutaneously according to a sliding scale. Alternative management, and that preferred in uncontrolled diabetics, consists of hourly blood glucose determinations with continuous administration of low-dose intravenous insulin.

Blood sugar monitoring should be continued until there is documentation of control. Intermediate-acting insulin may be prescribed when the oral carbohydrate intake is adequate. Patients whose blood sugar was controlled preoperatively with an oral hypoglycemic agent often do not require supplemental doses of insulin in the early postoperative period. They should, however, have periodic blood glucose determinations and regular insulin therapy, if indicated, to keep their blood sugar between 150 and 200 mg/dL. They may resume taking their oral hypoglycemic agents once they are on the appropriate diabetic diet.

Estrogen replacement therapy is recommended for patients who have undergone bilateral oophorectomy and who have no contraindications (abnormal liver function, acute vascular thrombosis, breast carcinoma) to its use. I begin estrogen replacement therapy when the patient resumes her regular diet. Replacement usually consists of conjugated equine estrogen, 0.625 mg, or transdermal estradiol, 0.05 mg, daily. Calcium supplementation is also prescribed to provide the patient with a daily intake of at least 1,000 mg of elemental calcium.

Feedings

Nausea and vomiting, which are common following a hysterectomy, may be caused by anesthetic agents and drugs, narcotic analgesics, pharyngeal stimulation, gastrointestinal distention or manipulation, sudden changes in position, hypotension, and/or pain. Control of nausea and vomiting is important in order to minimize the risk of tracheal aspiration and to prevent suture disruption, bleeding, and pain. The initial treatment of postoperative nausea and vomiting should consist of pain control, hydration, and maintenance of normal blood pressure. Persistent nausea and vomiting may require the administration of antiemetic medication.[1]

Surgical entry into the peritoneal cavity is usually followed by some degree of gastrointestinal dysfunction. This is more likely to be a problem after an abdominal hysterectomy than after a vaginal hysterectomy. Gastrointestinal dysfunction may also be caused by drugs, the patient's physical condition, the disease process, the complexity and length of the surgical procedure, contamination of the abdominal contents, and other factors. Patients who undergo a hysterectomy and have little bowel manipulation and no bowel surgery may be permitted to have clear liquids when there is no postoperative nausea or vomiting. Their diet may be advanced to include solid foods after the return of normal bowel sounds and the passage of flatus and/or feces. Constipation may be treated with gentle oral laxatives or rectal suppositories.

Ambulation

Emphasis should be placed on early ambulation, which prevents respiratory complications, promotes proper bowel function, and is considered to be important in lowering the risk of phlebitis, venous thrombosis, and pulmonary embolism. A patient who has an uncomplicated hysterectomy should be encouraged to sit on the side of her bed on the evening following surgery and to ambulate on the following day. The necessity for continued active ambulation should be emphasized daily and again when the patient is discharged from the hospital.

The time required for a patient to resume her normal activities depends on her physical condition, the surgical approach, the complexity of the surgical procedure, the presence or absence of postoperative complications, and the requirements of her daily routine. Walking in the house should be undertaken before walking outside; riding in a car should precede driving the car. Strenuous activities that significantly increase the intraabdominal pressure should be avoided in the early postoperative period to avoid stressing abdominal incisions and tissues in areas where any procedures might have been undertaken as treatment for pelvic organ prolapse.

Wound Care

Abdominal hysterectomy incisions should be covered by a sterile protective dressing before the patient leaves the operating room. If possible, abdominal drain sites should be dressed separately from the incision. All dressings should be examined frequently to determine their condition. If they become moist as a result of blood or serum, they should be changed and kept dry. If peritoneal fluid leaks from the skin incision, the wound should be examined for fascial dehiscence or evisceration. Such complications may require immediate surgical exploration and repair.

Abdominal dressings should be left in place for the first 48 to 72 hours to promote epithelialization and to protect the wound from the environment. Once epithelialization has occurred, there is no need for a dressing. The schedule for removing skin sutures, staples, or tape depends in part on the technique used to close the wound and will vary from surgeon to surgeon. Early removal of sutures or clips is often followed by the application of sterile adhesive strips that reduce the tension and tendency for the edges of the wound to separate.

Vaginal incisions require no special attention other than good personal hygiene. The patient should be advised against douching, using vaginal tampons, and having vaginal intercourse for at least 2 weeks following an uncomplicated hysterectomy and even longer if there has been an associated colporrhaphy.

Complications

Urinary Complications

Symptomatic urinary tract infections should be treated and the urine should be sterile before performing an elective hysterectomy. Patients with pelvic organ prolapse have an increased incidence of asymptomatic bacteriuria. Their urine should be rendered sterile prior to surgery to reduce the risk of postoperative infection of the urinary tract.

Urinary tract infections, the most common form of nosocomial infection, are usually caused by catheterization of the bladder.[2] The incidence of urinary tract infections increases with age and the number and duration of catheterizations. The likelihood of getting a urinary tract infection is directly related to the quality of catheter care. It is important to maintain a closed urinary collection system, to monitor the urine for bacterial colonization, and to keep indwelling bladder catheters in place for the shortest time possible.

There is no need to provide prophylactic medication to symptomatic patients with indwelling bladder catheters. Patients with catheters who develop symptomatic urinary tract infections should have a catheterized urine specimen sent for culture before therapy is begun. *Escherichia coli* is the cause of most urinary tract infections. Nitrofurantoin is ideal for the treatment of low-grade infections because it is specific for the treatment of urinary tract infections and will not mask other types of postoperative infections. Patients with more severe urinary tract infections may require parenteral antibiotic therapy. If this is the case, it should be remembered that hospital-acquired urinary tract infections may be resistant to commonly used antibiotics. Sensitivity studies will be of assistance in selecting the most appropriate antibiotic to be used.

Ureteral injury should be ruled out if flank pain coincides with onset of fever and/or the patient is unresponsive to antibiotic therapy. Ureteral obstruction requires ureteral catheterization, percutaneous nephrostomy, or surgical repair to preserve renal function. A genitourinary fistula should be suspected if urine drains from the vagina. Some of these fistulas will close spontaneously with placement of a ureteral and/or bladder catheter; others will require subsequent surgical repair.

Respiratory Complications

Patients with pulmonary disabilities are at increased risk for developing postoperative respiratory complications. Additional risk factors include cigarette smoking, advanced age, obesity, and malnutrition. Measures should be undertaken to improve pulmonary function before allowing these patients to undergo elective surgery. Respiratory complications are more likely to occur after abdominal hysterectomies than after vaginal hysterectomies.

Respiratory complications are minimized by maintaining a patent airway, preventing tracheal aspiration, judicious use of narcotic analgesics, frequent turning and deep breathing, the aggressive use of incentive spirometry, and early ambulation. Respiratory failure is associated with sweating, tachycardia, hypertension, and evidence of hypoxia. The diagnosis is confirmed by finding an increased $PaCO_2$. Treatment includes clearing the airway and providing oxygen, bronchodilators, chest physical therapy, antibiotics for bacterial pneumonia, and possible ventilatory support.

Atelectasis is the most frequent postoperative respiratory complication. It occurs in 10% to 15% of patients without risk factors who have lower abdominal surgery.[11] The diagnosis is suggested by finding basilar rales, absent or bronchial breath sounds, a productive cough, fever, and leukocytosis. Atelectasis may be complicated by the development of pneumonia.

Pneumonia is the third most common nosocomial infection and is the one most likely to cause death.[2] It is usually manifested by fever, cough, a productive sputum, and, on chest radiograph, a pulmonary infiltrate. Bacteria gain access to the lungs as a result of aspiration of oropharyngeal or gastric secretions, by inhaling bacteria laden aerosols, or by hematogenous spread from other infections within the body. The presence of *Staphylococcus aureus* or *E. coli* in the sputum suggests a hospital-acquired infection. Same-day surgery may make community-acquired pathogens (*Streptococcus pneumoniae*, *Haemophilus influenzae*, *Mycoplasma*, and *Legionella*) more common. Therapy consists of broad-spectrum antibiotic (eg, cefazolin and gentamicin) therapy, hydration, careful airway management, coughing, deep-breathing exercises, chest physical therapy, the use of incentive spirometry, and, in selected cases, assisted ventilation.

Pulmonary embolism is an acute, life-threatening pulmonary disorder. The source of the emboli is usually deep leg veins. Physical findings include dyspnea, tachypnea, rales, hypoxemia, and syncope or shock. An electrocardiogram usually shows sinus tachycardia, T-wave inversion, and nonspecific ST segment changes. The evaluation should include a chest radiograph and perfusion lung scan. A normal perfusion lung scan is strong evidence against the diagnosis of pulmonary embolism. If the perfusion lung scan is equivocal, pulmonary arteriography should be considered. Treatment of pulmonary embolism consists of oxygen administration, hydration, and rapid intravenous heparinization. Intravenous fibrinolytic (streptokinase or urokinase) therapy may be used in patients who are extremely symptomatic or have mild hemodynamic instability. Such therapy, however, has not been shown to be superior to anticoagulation therapy, and streptokinase may be associated with severe allergic reactions. If the patient experiences a massive pulmonary embolism and anticoagulation therapy is contraindicated, surgical embolectomy may be lifesaving. Vena caval filters are recommended for patients who have recurrent emboli in spite of adequate anticoagulation.[2,12]

Cardiovascular Complications

Postoperative hypotension is usually due to uncontrollable bleeding, inadequate fluid or blood replacement, depression of the cardiovascular system by anesthetic agents or drugs, or a cardiovascular catastrophe (eg, myocardial infarction or pulmonary embolism). Oxygen and fluid administration are recommended during attempts to make a definitive diagnosis. Vasopressors may be required.

Posthysterectomy arterial hemorrhage is most often due to bleeding from an ovarian artery or from a branch of the anterior division of the internal iliac artery. Appropriate intravenous therapy and pain relief should be provided. If the bleeding cannot be controlled by vaginal examination and suture placement, I favor selective arterial embolization. If this is not available, exploratory laparotomy with ligation of the bleeding vessel and/or hypogastric artery ligation may be required. Packing is usually more effective for venous hemorrhage than attempts at suture ligation. Delayed postoperative hemorrhage is usually due to tissue necrosis, infection, or suture absorption.

Postoperative hypertension may be due to pain, agitation, hypothermia, hypercapnia, or hypoxia. Although usually self-limited, it may be complicated by pulmonary edema, heart failure, cardiac arrhythmia, or stroke. It should be treated by administering oxygen and relieving pain. If the condition persists, drug therapy may be required.

Ventricular arrhythmias are treated with lidocaine infusions and, if necessary, direct current shock. Atrial arrhythmias are treated with vagal stimulation or by administering propranolol. The development of a postoperative cardiac arrhythmia suggests the possibility of occult heart disease.

Deep venous thrombosis occurs in approximately 7% of patients undergoing vaginal hysterectomy and 13% undergoing abdominal hysterectomy for benign disorders. Approximately 1% of those patients will experience fatal pulmonary embolism.[13] The risk factors include obesity, aging, immobility, malignancy, trauma, surgery, and myocardial infarction. The causes of thrombophlebitis and deep venous thrombosis include venous stasis, hypercoagulability, and endothelial damage (Virchow's triad). The clinical findings of thrombophlebitis and venous thrombosis are nonspecific (50% false positive). They include pain (40%), pitting edema, and blanching of the skin (phlegmasia alba dolens).[12] The left iliac vein is more often involved than the right iliac vein. Diagnostic studies are of limited value below the knee. Venography is the most accurate method of confirming the diagnosis and determining the extent of thrombosis. Doppler has a sensitivity of over 90% and a specificity of 5% to 10% for popliteal, femoral, and iliac thromboses.[12]

Prophylaxis for thrombophlebitis and venous thrombosis includes early ambulation, low-dose heparin (5,000 units 2 hours before surgery and every 12 hours until fully ambulatory), and the use of intermittent pneumatic compression stockings on the lower extremities. Treatment of thrombophlebitis and venous thrombosis is aimed at minimizing the risk of pulmonary embolism, limiting further thrombosis, and facilitating the resolution of existing thrombi. The affected patient should be started on sufficient heparin to maintain the activated partial thromboplastin time at a level that is 1.5 to 2 times normal control values, and anticoagulation should be continued with warfarin in a sufficient dosage to maintain the prothrombin time at 1.3 to 1.5 times normal control values for up to 3 months.[11] Fibrinolytic therapy has not been shown to be superior to anticoagulant therapy in the treatment of deep venous thrombosis.

Contamination of an intravenous line may cause superficial thrombophlebitis and, on rare occasion, a septicemia. Common nosocomial pathogens include *Klebsiella, Enterobacter*, and *Serratia*. This complication is minimized by using aseptic placement techniques and by changing the intravenous line every 48 to 72 hours. When superficial thrombophlebitis is due to a contaminated intravenous line, it usually requires removal of the intravenous line, elevation of the extremity, and the application of warm compresses. Antibiotic therapy may be indicated if there is a septicemia. Suppurative thrombophlebitis, unresponsive to antibiotic therapy, may require surgical excision of the involved segment of the vein.

Septic pelvic thrombophlebitis is an uncommon complication of a hysterectomy, unless the hysterectomy is performed during or soon after pregnancy. The diagnosis must be entertained when a patient who is being treated for pelvic cellulitis does not respond to antibiotic therapy. The diagnosis is aided by ultrasound or computerized tomograms of the pelvis. Patients with septic pelvic thrombophlebitis usually respond dramatically to heparin therapy.

Gastrointestinal Complications

A paralytic ileus develops when air is trapped in the small intestine as a result of hypoactivity of the bowel or closure of the ileocecal valve. Although a paralytic ileus may be caused by manipulation of the abdominal contents, it is more likely to be the result of electrolyte imbalance, ketoacidosis, gastrointestinal injury, uremia, or sepsis. The patient develops abdominal distention, nausea, and vomiting; bowel sounds are absent. Abdominal radiographs show air in the small intestine and usually in the colon. Initial treatment should be conservative. Oral intake is withheld pending evidence of bowel function; appropriate intravenous fluid and electrolyte therapy is ordered and, if the patient complains of vomiting and abdominal distention, nasogastric suction may be used.

Intestinal obstructions usually occur after the fourth or fifth postoperative day. Small bowel obstruction is associated with cramping abdominal pain and vomiting. Large bowel obstruction is more likely to be associated with abdominal distention and pain in the lower abdomen. Vomiting is less likely to occur with large bowel obstruction. Most intestinal obstructions are caused by adhesions or hernias; some are the result of intrinsic disease, intussusception of the bowel, or volvulus. Bowel sounds are initially active, with rushes, but in time they may become hypoactive. Rebound abdominal tenderness suggests an inflammatory process or strangulation of the bowel. Abdominal radiographs show dilated loops of bowel, usually with air-filled levels proximal to the obstruction and no distal gas pattern. Treatment consists of withholding oral intake, administering intravenous fluid and electrolyte therapy, intestinal intubation, and antibiotic therapy for sepsis. In mechanical bowel obstruction, it is important to recognize the need for early surgical exploration.

Wound Complications

Hysterectomies involve an incision into the vagina and are, therefore, classified according to the American College of Surgeons as "clean-contaminated" cases. The incidence of wound infections in this category of cases is approximately 10%.[2]

Wound infections are the third most common nosocomial infection[2] and usually occur within 2 weeks of surgery. Risk factors for abdominal wound infections include obesity, advancing age, preoperative hospitalization, prolonged surgical procedure, sepsis elsewhere in the body, and medical or pharmacologic conditions compromising the immune system. Wound infections are manifested by erythema, edema, tenderness, and drainage. Abdominal wound infections that follow a hysterectomy are commonly caused by *S. aureus* and aerobic gram-negative rods or by organisms found at the vaginal cuff, frequently the anaerobes. The primary treatment of abdominal wound infections is surgical drainage. Necrotizing infections should be treated by wide excision of all involved tissues. Antibiotic therapy is helpful if there is significant cellulitis about the edges of the wound or evidence of systemic infection.[2]

Pelvic Cellulitis

The incidence of pelvic cellulitis following hysterectomy depends on the risk factors for the patient population, the use of prophylactic antibiotics, and the indications for surgery. Risk factors include reproductive age, low socioeconomic status, and duration of the operative procedure.[14] Once other sources of infection have been excluded, the diagnostic criteria include fever, pelvic pain, and vaginal cuff tenderness and induration. Ultrasound and computerized tomographic scanning of the pelvis may be helpful in confirming the diagnosis. Pelvic cellulitis and pelvic abscess are usually polymicrobial (aerobic and anerobic organisms) in origin. Three percent of cases may develop a pelvic abscess, which is more common after vaginal than after abdominal hysterectomies. Patients with inflammatory bowel disease (appendicitis, Crohn's disease, or diverticulitis) are at increased risk for developing postoperative pelvic abscesses, 75% of which are vaginal cuff abscesses and 25% of which are adnexal abscesses.[14] Pelvic abscesses are more commonly anaerobic in origin and should be treated with broad-spectrum antibiotics (clindamycin/gentamicin, cefoxitin, ceftizoxime, etc). The treatment of a pelvic abscess includes broad-spectrum antibiotic coverage that ensures good anaerobic coverage (clindamycin, metronidazole) and, perhaps, surgical drainage. A tuboovarian abscess may require exploratory laparotomy and adnexectomy.

Drug Fever

Drug fevers are allergic reactions. The promptness with which they occur depends on previous exposure to the same or related drugs. Although the patient usually appears well, her fever pattern may be remittent (60%; a variable but elevated daily temperature), intermittent (30%; fever with temperature returning to normal daily), or hectic (10%; intermittent or remittent fever with 1.4°C difference between highest and lowest values). Antibiotics (penicillins and cephalosporins) are responsible for the largest number of drug fevers.[15] The diagnosis is one of exclusion. Drug fevers usually subside within 48 to 72 hours of discontinuing the responsible drug.

Discharge from Hospital and Follow-Up

Patients should plan for their convalescence prior to being admitted for their surgery by arranging for help for their personal and medical needs. Unforeseen complications during their hospitalization may require the services of a home health care agency. The hospital staff is usually knowledgeable of community resources.

Patients should not be discharged from the hospital until it is medically advisable to do so. Patients undergoing a vaginal hysterectomy usually experience quicker return of normal physiologic functions and less pain than do patients undergoing an abdominal hysterectomy. Therefore, it is the operative approach and the presence or absence of significant operative and postoperative complications that determine the length of hospitalization.

It is helpful to give each patient verbal and printed discharge instruction (Table 10.3). In addition to a prescription for pain control, prescriptions may be needed for antibiotics, hormone replacement, or necessary daily medications. All patients should be told to call their physician's office to report complications or concerns. The timing of their office visits will depend on their individual needs.

Table 10.3 Suggested Discharge Instructions for Patients following Hysterectomy

1. Continue hospital-like routine for the first 1 or 2 days
2. Limit strenuous activities (eg, climbing steps, heavy housework, lifting)
3. May shower or bathe as desired
4. Avoid douches, tampons, intercourse for at least 2 weeks
5. Light bloody or brown vaginal discharge will persist for a couple of weeks; report any significant bright red bleeding
6. Avoid constipation; use gentle laxatives, if needed
7. Report fevers >101 °F
8. Call your surgeon if there are complications or concerns
9. Schedule office visit in 6 weeks or earlier if instructed to do so
10. Do not return to work until you obtain your surgeon's approval

References

1. Tewes PA, Taylor DR, Bourke DL: Postoperative pain management, in Breslow MJ, Miller CF, Rogers MC (eds): *Perioperative Management*. St. Louis, CV Mosby, 1990, pp 164–179.
2. Committee on Pre and Postoperative Care, American College of Surgeons: *Care of the Surgical Patient, vol 1: Elective Care*. New York, Scientific American, Inc, 1988.
3. Rosenfeld BA, Miller CF: Commonly encountered recovery room problems, in Breslow MJ, Miller CF, Rogers MC (eds): *Perioperative Management*. St. Louis, CV Mosby, 1990, pp 148–163.
4. US Department of Health and Human Services, National Institutes of Health: National Blood Resource Education Program, publication No. 89-297a. Washington, DC, US Government Printing Office, 1989.
5. Muller MC: Anesthesia for the patient with renal dysfunction. *Int Anaesthesiol Clin* 1984;22:169–187.
6. Fritsche CM, Hebert LA, Lemann J Jr: Water, electrolyte and acid-base metabolism, in Thompson JD, Rock JR (eds): *TeLinde's Operative Gynecology*, ed 7. Philadelphia, JB Lippincott, 1992, pp 123–150.
7. Donovan M, Dillon P, McGuire L: Incidence and characteristics of pain in a sample of medical-surgical patients. *Pain* 1987;30:69–78.
8. Kaplan R, Goldofsky S, Claudio M: Pain management, in Frost EAM, Goldiner PL, Bryan-Brown C (eds): *Postanesthetic Care*. Norwalk, CT, Appleton and Lange, 1990, pp 43–62.
9. Soper DE, Yarwood R: Single dose antimicrobial prophylaxis for vaginal hysterectomies. *Obstet Gynecol* 1987;69:879–882.
10. Baker VV: Postoperative consideration of the gynecology patient, in Shingleton HM, Hurt WG (eds): *Postreproductive Gynecology*. New York, Churchill Livingstone, 1990, pp 517–528.
11. Droegemueller W: Postoperative complications, in Herbst AL, Mishell DR Jr, Stenchever MA, et al (eds): *Comprehensive Gynecology*, ed 2. St. Louis, Mosby–Year Book, 1992, pp 753–797.
12. Greenfield LJ: Complications of venous thrombosis and pulmonary embo-

lism, in Greenfield LJ (ed): *Complications in Surgery and Trauma*, ed 2. Philadelphia, JB Lippincott, 1990, pp 430–445.
13. Walsh JJ, Bonnar J, Wright FW: A study of pulmonary embolism and deep leg vein thrombosis after major gynaecological surgery using labelled fibrinogen-phlebography and lung scanning. *J Obstet Gynaecol Br Commonw* 1974;81:311–316.
14. Shapiro M, Munoz A, Tager IB, et al: Risk factors for infection at the operative site after abdominal and vaginal hysterectomy. *N Engl J Med* 1982;307:1661–1666.
15. Mackowiak PA, LeMaistre CF: Drug fever: A critical appraisal of conventional concepts. *Ann Intern Med* 1987;106:728–733.

Chapter **11**

Psychosocial Aspects of Hysterectomy

Renate H. Rosenthal, PhD, and Frank W. Ling, MD

From a physician's standpoint, a hysterectomy is only one in a series of procedures that are done for well-chosen medical indications. There is little if any emotional investment in the procedure, because it is viewed as a necessary medical intervention on behalf of the patient's welfare. The process of deciding to perform a hysterectomy has been a logical, calculated, step-by-step progression. In distinct contrast to this, for the patient undergoing hysterectomy, the procedure represents a single, unique experience that potentially alters how she thinks about herself and/or how she thinks she is perceived by others. Not only must the patient face the risks of anesthesia, intra- and postoperative complications, and a potentially extended rehabilitation, she must also, in the case of hysterectomy with or without oophorectomy, possibly have to reevaluate her sense of identity.

With the loss of the uterus, the patient must deal with the inability to menstruate and procreate, to calmly accept changes in overt signs of femininity. Paradoxically, the hysterectomy is performed to improve quality of life, but the circumstances surrounding the procedure may very well, if not addressed directly, leave the patient more dysfunctional than she had been preoperatively. Massler and Devansan[1] have written that the magnitude of any emotional response to a physical assault on a person's body is proportional to the degree to which the person is emotionally invested in that body part. Specifically, female parts that are most vulnerable are the breasts, genitalia, face, hair, and abdominal wall. Added to this are the common emotional responses to surgery of any type (vulnerability, anxiety, dependency, and grief). These emotional responses result in the very real potential for psychosocial maladjustment after hysterectomy. It is only with active preventative intervention on the part of the health care system preoperatively as well as close scrutiny postoperatively that a poor psychosocial outcome can be minimized.

Because the patient of today takes a more active role in the decision-making process regarding hysterectomy, the sense of loss of control over her own fate is not as significant as it once was. There is clearly, however, the very real loss of control in the sense that someone else must perform the operation.

Emotional Issues as the Underlying Cause of Gynecologic Complaints

Historic Perspective

The ancient Egyptians postulated a simple causal relationship between the uterus and some women's puzzling physical and emotional complaints, now referred to as hysteria. These behaviors were ascribed to the syndrome of the "wandering uterus." Medical treatment consisted of efforts to return the wandering womb to its correct location. To accomplish this goal, women were given noxious medicines to inhale or to ingest, and sweet-smelling substances were placed between the patient's legs to attract the uterus back to where it belonged.[2] Contemporary psychology might view this approach as a behavioral intervention, designed to discourage "hysterical" symptoms and minimize secondary gain by administering aversive consequences to the behavior in question.

The French neurologist Charcot viewed women's unexplained somatic or emotional distress as an indication of psychosocial trauma. He treated these patients with hypnosis, with promising results. In the trance, the women revealed information about issues they were unable to talk about while fully awake; often these were sexual in nature. Sigmund Freud studied with Charcot. The concept of unconscious motivation and unconscious conflict intrigued Freud and served as the initial inspiration for his psychoanalytic theory.

Briquet's Syndrome (Somatization Disorder)

The syndrome of multiple somatic complaints without a demonstrable organic basis continued to be referred to as "hysteria" until the 1970s. In an effort to delineate the diagnosis and avoid the pejorative term "hysteria," Samuel Guze and his colleagues coined the term "Briquet's syndrome."[3] The disorder became the subject of extensive scientific research. There are now numerous well-controlled studies that show a link between Briquet's disorder (also known as Briquet's somatization syndrome) in women and antisocial personality disorder (sociopathy) in their male first-degree relatives.[4] There appears to be a significant genetic component to both disorders. The *Diagnostic and Statistical Manual of Mental Disorders* (ed 3, revised)[5] uses the term "Somatization Disorder" to describe Briquet's syndrome. The two concepts overlap significantly. To justify the diagnosis, a patient must have a chronic or recurrent disorder, characterized by many physical complaints, beginning before the age of 30 and persisting for several years. There may or may not be physical findings. The medical history is dramatic, vague, and very complicated. If there is organic pathology, the patient's complaints and invalidism are much in excess of what would normally be expected. Often the patient reports medically unexplained problems in multiple organ systems. She describes her discomfort in very colorful and exaggerated terms, resists reassurance, and desires medications, diagnostic tests, and surgery.

Ballinger[6] found that psychiatric morbidity was notably high in patients whose chief complaint was menorrhagia, particularly in those women who ultimately had hysterectomies. Barker[7] found that women whose pathology report after surgery failed to reveal significant gynecologic disease were five times more likely to have had a psychiatric history ($p < .005$) than were patients who had identifiable gynecologic disease. One may conjecture that the former patients described their symptoms in particularly florid and compelling ways. The patient's subjective distress, rather than extent of disease or dysfunction, often determines whether or not surgery is performed. Martin et al[8] prospectively studied 49 randomly selected women who received hysterectomies for reasons other than cancer and found 57% to be psychiatrically ill: 27% satisfied the diagnostic criteria for Briquet's syndrome and 18% had primary depression. A frequency of Briquet's somatization syndrome of 27% is in great excess of the age-adjusted estimate of 2.4% of the general female population. However, the prevalence of 18% for primary depression is close to other reports of the life-time morbidity for depression in women.[9]

Somatic symptoms are likely to flare up in times of emotional stress, but the somatizing patient has little or no awareness of this connection and takes strong offense at the suggestion that emotions may play a part in her discomfort. She looks to the medical profession to provide help and support for problems that often are rooted in psychosocial difficulties.

Because of their dramatic presentation and their insistence on "having something done" to feel better, somatization disorder patients are at increased risk for unnecessary surgery to alleviate their symptoms. This seems to apply particularly to abdominal surgery because the complaints often include painful menstruation, irregular periods, excessive menstrual bleeding, dyspareunia, and abdominal pain (Figure 11.1). Martin et al,[10] in a prospective study of 44 patients, found that 39 reported relief or improvement in symptoms at 1-year follow-up. All five denying improvement fulfilled the diagnostic criteria for Briquet's somatization syndrome preoperatively.

It should be noted that a total of 13 patients in this study were diagnosed as having Briquet's disorder preoperatively. Of these 13, eight improved after surgery. However, whereas 38% of the Briquet's patients reported an unsatisfactory outcome of surgery, none of the 36 non-Briquet's patients did. These proportions are significant at $p = .0007$ by Fisher's exact probability test.

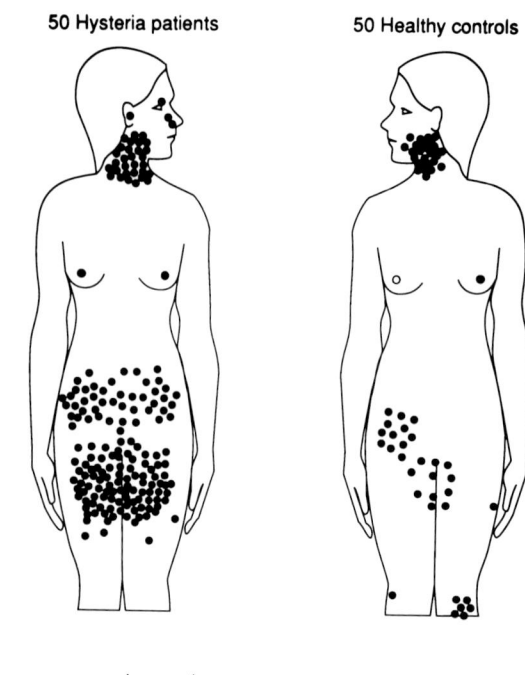

Figure 11.1 Reprinted, by permission, from Cohen et al: JAMA 1953; 151:977–986.

● = 1 operation

Perley and Guze[11] tabulated the frequency of somatic complaints in patients with Briquet's disorder: 80% suffered from abdominal pain, 48% reported excessive menstrual bleeding, and another 48% had irregular menses. Sexual indifference was reported by 44%, and 52% had dyspareunia. The list of other physical problems reported by these patients is truly impressive and comprises a total of 59 complaint categories. The dysfunctions involved every system of the body (Table 11.1). In the absence of other information, a plethora of somatic complaints should raise a "red flag" for suspicion of somatization disorder.[12,13]

In a retrospective study, Waldemar et al[14] found that somatization disorder could have been the underlying cause for hysterectomy as well as for complaints resulting in neurologic consultation. Among women discharged from a neurologic service with no objective neurologic findings, the incidence of hysterectomy was 14% compared with a 5.4% incidence of hysterectomy among women who had organic neurologic disease. Among the pathologic specimens in the group without demonstrable neurologic findings, 22 of 30 were normal. Waldemar et al concluded that the complaints that led to hysterectomy could very well have been better served by the combined efforts of a psychiatrist and primary care physician. Preoperative awareness of this possibility could reduce the number of hysterectomies performed for symptoms that do not resolve postoperatively.

Gynecologic surgeons should be particularly sensitized to the po-

Table 11.1. Frequency of Symptoms in Hysteria

Symptom	%	Symptom	%
Dyspnea	72	Dysuria	44
Palpitation	60	Urinary retention	8
Chest pain	72	Dysmenorrhea (premarital only)	4
Dizziness	84	Dysmenorrhea (prepregnancy only)	8
Headache	80	Dysmenorrhea (other)	48
Anxiety attacks	64	Menstrual irregularity	48
Fatigue	84	Excessive menstrual bleeding	48
Blindness	20	Sexual indifference	44
Paralysis	12	Frigidity (absence of orgasm)	24
Anesthesia	32	Dyspareunia	52
Aphonia	44	Back pain	88
Lump in throat	28	Joint pain	84
Fits or convulsions	20	Extremity pain	84
Faints	56	Burning pains in rectum, vagina, mouth	28
Unconsciousness	16	Other bodily pain	36
Amnesia	8	Depressed feelings	64
Visual blurring	64	Phobias	48
Visual hallucination	12	Vomiting all nine months of pregnancy	20
Deafness	4	Nervous	92
Olfactory hallucination	16	Had to quit working because felt bad	44
Weight loss	28	Trouble doing anything because felt bad	72
Sudden fluctuations in weight	16	Cried a lot	60
Anorexia	60	Felt life was hopeless	28
Nausea	80	Always sickly (most of life)	40
Vomiting	32	Thought of dying	48
Abdominal pain	80	Wanted to die	36
Abdominal bloating	68	Thought of suicide	28
Food intolerances	48	Attempted suicide	12
Diarrhea	20	Weakness	84
Constipation	64		

Reprinted, by permission, from Perley M, Guze SB: Hysteria: The stability and usefulness of clinical criteria. *N Engl J Med* 1962;266:421–426.

tential outcome in patients being considered for hysterectomy when either no specific pathology is found during the preoperative work-up or the surgical specimen is normal. Bang et al[15] reported a prospective series in which there was a higher incidence of psychosomatic symptoms among patients in whom the hysterectomy specimen did not satisfactorily explain the preoperative symptoms.

According to Dennerstein and van Hall,[16] the hysterectomy rate in the United States is twice that in the United Kingdom. Given the frequency of "benign" pelvic complaints in women with Briquet's disorder, it is possible that more Briquet's patients are operated on in this country.

Clinical Approach to the Somatizing Patient

Patients with Briquet's (somatization) disorder tend to express emotional conflict in terms of physical complaints. They often seem to lack the ability to articulate their feelings, to analyze their situation with detachment, and to design a course of action for themselves to alleviate their emotional pain. Rather, they seek help and comfort from members of the medical profession, reciting their physical complaints in great detail. This inability to put feelings into words is known as "alexithymia." The concept means "no words for mood" and was first introduced by Sifneos[17] in 1973. The ability to communicate feelings verbally is largely a learned behavior. Children who are exposed to physical illness and pain behavior in their homes are more likely to exhibit somatization.[18,19] Children raised in homes where verbal expression of feelings is not modeled, is discouraged, or even is punished often also are subject to physical, emotional, or sexual abuse. Given the strong familial link between somatization and sociopathy, one may safely conjecture that heredity as well as dysfunctional family environment play an important role in molding the coping style of women with somatization disorder.

These patients' symptom presentation often is so dramatic, and their plea for medical help is so heartfelt, that they tend to bring about strong emotions in their caregiver. An initial desire to rush to the patient's rescue often is followed by resentment if the interventions have not brought relief. The patient, in turn, experiences yet another bout of being "let down" by someone she had trusted. This often is the beginning of an extended search for physicians who will "fix" the patient's physical problem. In the natural course of events, many of these women ultimately present with chronic pelvic pain that is unresponsive to medical and nonsurgical intervention.

Traditional insight-oriented psychotherapy rarely appeals to patients with somatization disorder. However, many can be taught, over time, to view their symptoms with more detachment and to entertain the possibility that emotional stress may be making their symptoms worse. In our experience, most of the initial work in this regard must take place in the physician's office, rather than by referring a troublesome patient prematurely to a mental health professional. In the absence of compelling physical findings that would explain the patient's discomfort, we often take a "good news—bad news" approach:

"I have examined you and I have looked at all the tests and x-rays we have done. I have good news and bad news: The *good* news is that there is nothing going on that is dangerous or would require an operation right now. There is no evidence that you have any type of major disease. The *bad* news is that you obviously are in quite a bit of discomfort and I am taking this very seriously. I'm not in any way saying that this is all in your head. Your discomfort is very real. What I *am* saying is that sometimes tension and stress can cause all kinds of physical symptoms. You have heard of tension headaches. You may even have had some. Those are *real* headaches. The pain is real. The *source* of the pain, however, is tension and stress. We know for a fact that some people are more likely to develop pain and discomfort when they are under stress. People can come down with stress-related symptoms in any part of the body. I'm not sure yet what all is going on in your life, but I suspect that there are quite a few things that are burdening you more than you know."

At this point, the patient may reveal some of her problems. If she fails to do so, the following instructions may be helpful:

"Sometimes it takes a while before we realize that something is really getting next to us and bothering us. All we notice is the physical pain. I would like to see you again not too long from now and maybe you can come up with some connections in the meantime. I know you are very concerned about your health and I am not ignoring your complaint. I'm planning to keep a good eye on what's going on."

Over time, referral to a psychologist or psychiatrist may be acceptable to the patient, especially once she has made a connection between her life stresses and her discomfort. In the interim, emergency room visits and "doctor shopping" must be strongly discouraged. Ford has provided an excellent practical discussion of diagnostic and management issues of somatizing patients.[20]

Emotional Problems as the Consequence of Gynecologic Problems

Reproductive function is a major issue for most women. Hollender[21] pointed out that the ability to have children, even if it is never used, is important for the woman's self-image. However, nulliparity, by itself, has not been shown to be a major risk factor for emotional problems after hysterectomy, especially if the patient is in a supportive, stable relationship.[7]

Although some women feel menstruation is a "curse" and are delighted to be spared the monthly ordeal after hysterectomy, others see their menses as an integral part of their womanhood. Drellich and Bieber[22] interviewed 23 women who had recently undergone hysterectomies. The majority saw menstrual periods as a necessary and valuable function and viewed their termination with regret. This is true even for women who had suffered from significant dysmenorrhea. The menstrual cycle was viewed as a kind of "psychologic metronome" that lends predictability to life's routines. Also, several women felt that menstruation serves a cleaning function, ridding the body of waste, and commented on feeling energized and refreshed after their monthly cycle. These women experienced cessation of menses as a loss.

Depression and Anxiety

Lindemann[23] described a postoperative syndrome that resembled an agitated depression and that followed hysterectomy more often than surgery of the upper abdomen. Richards[24,25] reported a posthysterectomy syndrome characterized by postoperative depression and multiple somatic complaints. Hollender[21] reported similar findings: Almost twice as many women were admitted to a psychiatric hospital following pelvic operations as following all other types of surgery. Agitated depression was the most common presentation. In contrast, Bragg,[26] comparing later psychiatric hospital admissions rates of 1,601 hysterectomy patients and 1,162 cholecystectomy controls, failed to find significant differences. There is disagreement in the literature about the frequency of depression as a complication of hysterectomy. The criteria used to define depression vary; so does the follow-up period after surgery. Much of the information was collected retrospectively and, as a result, suffers on a methodologic basis.

A further complication is that a significant number of patients seem to have preexisting psychiatric disturbance, most commonly, Briquet's somatization syndrome.[8,10] Persistent features of this disorder, including recurrent pains, nervousness, depression, and sexual and marital problems, can occur both before and after surgery. There is no way to assess how many of the patients suffering from "posthysterectomy syndrome" actually had preexisting problems that set the stage for the symptoms attributed to the surgery. Therein lies the problem with retrospectively collected data. For example, in a retrospective study, Moore and Tolley[27] found that 32% of patients were depressed 6 months after surgery, as measured by the Zung Self-Rating Depression Scale (SDS). However, the majority of these women were depressed before they had the operation.

Martin et al[10] showed a decrease in Zung SDS scores 1 year after hysterectomy. In this prospective study, of the 14 women who had clinically significant depression scores (SDS greater than 50) prior to surgery, seven had normal SDS scores at follow-up. This difference was significant at Chi square = 9.50 ($p < .005$). Meikle and Brody[28] studied 55 hysterectomy, 60 tubal ligation, and 38 cholecystectomy patients prospectively, using the 65-item Profile of Mood States (POMS) questionnaire.[29] Hysterectomy did not result in a greater degree of mood disturbance. Similar results were reported by Hampton and Tarnasky.[30] Gath et al[31] found, in a prospective study of 156 women with menorrhagia of benign origin, that the extent of psychiatric problems in the patients exceeded what one would expect in the general population. However, after the surgery, psychiatric symptoms decreased from 58% of patients to 29% at 18-month follow-up, as assessed on the POMS, among other measures. Sexual adjustment and social functioning were also improved. There was a significant excess of marital problems in women who had psychiatric symptoms before and/or after the surgery.

A more recent study by Lalinec-Michaud et al[32] compared women undergoing hysterectomy, different abdominal operations, and cholecystectomy. One year after surgery, the hysterectomy group did not differ significantly from the other groups on depression scores, postoperative general adjustment, sexual satisfaction, or relationship to partner. However, patients in all three groups experienced a slight increase in depression scores up to 1 month after surgery. As time went on, depression decreased. In the hysterectomy group, almost half of the women with elevated depression scores postoperatively had scored high on depression prior to the surgery. There was no difference in depression for vaginal versus abdominal hysterectomy. The most consistent finding in studies of postoperative depression seems to be that the best predictor is a history of depression earlier in the patient's life. There is no consensus about a peak period. Patients whose partners had a negative attitude about the operation seem to be at higher risk for depression.[33]

Anxiety and depression should not be viewed as distinct and separate disorders. Recent evidence suggests that there is considerable overlap in symptomatology between patients who complain primarily of dysphoria and those who complain primarily of anxious mood.[34] There is little information about anxiety in relation to hysterectomy for reasons other than cancer. Drellich and Bieber[22,35] noted the occurrence of significant anxiety in the women they studied. However, their patients were drawn from an oncology setting. Much of their anxiety related to fear of disfigurement and disability. One may conjecture that some of the common postoperative complaints of "hot flushes," headaches, insomnia, and dizziness are anxiety related,[25,36] perhaps in women who are prone to somatization.

The most recent studies with regard to posthysterectomy psychological changes are more methodologically sound and have found little evidence that hysterectomy leads to depression. As mentioned, in Gath et al's study of 156 women,[31,37] postoperative psychopathology was best predicted by preoperative psychopathology. Sixty percent of those who had a psychiatric diagnosis before their hysterectomy no longer had a diagnosis when followed 18 months later. The majority of cases had been diagnosed with mild depression or anxiety. Lack of uterine pathology in the surgical specimen, age, oophorectomy, or other surgical factors were not associated with postoperative diagnosis of psychopathology.

Hollender[21] suggested that vaginal surgery can rekindle unresolved emotional conflicts. A recent report suggests that hysterectomy may reactivate psychic trauma of a sexual nature that had been successfully repressed, bringing about symptoms of a delayed posttraumatic stress disorder. Hendricks-Matthews[38] cited a case of a 33-year-old woman who had been raped at knife-point 12 years prior. At that time, she had experienced feelings of being different and isolated from other women, but had been relatively successful at repressing her trauma until she faced the prospect of having a hysterectomy. She experienced acute panic attacks and feelings of depersonalization prior to the scheduled date of the operation. She stated she felt as if she were to be "raped all over again."

Although this report is based only on one case, it is not an isolated instance. The present authors are familiar with several patients who experienced "flashbacks" of sexual trauma following gynecologic surgery.

Following hysterectomy, one patient became severely depressed and preoccupied with emotional and sexual abuse that had taken place in her childhood and adolescence. This woman had been able to repress her problems for many years and never sought psychiatric help. She also likened her hysterectomy to "being raped all over again."

A second patient from our practice developed "flashbacks" and nightmares following gynecologic surgery for vulvar intraepithelial neoplasia. This woman was well known to one of the authors (RHR) because she had sought counseling for marital problems more than a decade prior to the gynecologic surgery. The patient's first husband, whom she later divorced, had insisted on sadomasochistic sexual practices. This went on throughout the years of their marriage and caused the patient significant physical and emotional distress. The patient finally obtained a divorce. Several years later, she remarried and described her second husband as kind, gentle, caring, and considerate. She felt their sex life was very good until she had gynecologic surgery. Then, she suddenly began to vividly relive the sadomasochistic traumatic experiences she had had with her first husband. She felt anxious and humiliated, had nightmares, could not stand to be touched, stated she hated the idea of sex, and urged her new husband to go and find someone who would be a better sexual partner for him since she could no longer please him.

All three cases illustrate the fact that recollections of past traumatic experiences may be rekindled by events seemingly far removed from the original trauma. For this reason, it is very important to include inquiry about previous sexual trauma in any sexual history. If there has been abuse or trauma, the woman will require more emotional support and closer follow-up than is routinely given. Women who have been abused seem to be at higher risk for developing chronic pain syndromes.

A Canadian study[39] demonstrated that there can be a strong culturally based response to hysterectomy. Among 152 women who underwent hysterectomy, prospectively obtained questionnaires showed that women of European origin had greater postoperative regret and had greater difficulty adjusting after hysterectomy than did their counterparts who were French-Canadian or English-Canadian. Significant contributing factors included level of education (fewer problems with more education), family structure (more problems when the maternal role was highly emphasized), and immigration status (more problems when there was a lack of social integration). Physician and patient awareness of the potential effects of such factors can help minimize the psychologic morbidity associated with this operation.

In an Australian study, Ryan et al[40] found, in following 90 women after hysterectomy up to 14 months, that there was no evidence of greater psychological distress. Specifically, there was a 55% prevalence of preoperative psychopathology that was reduced to 31.7% postoperatively. This study also addressed the possibility that participation in the research process could have affected patient outcome—that is, that a patient could do better as a reflection of greater interest and concern on the part of the researcher. This was not found to be the case, however.

Behavior Problems

Hackett and Weisman[41] viewed the psychological aspects of surgery from three vantage points. On an intrapersonal level, how the patient perceives herself and her own body parts is a critical factor. A second level is the people surrounding the patient (eg, family, friends, and the health care team). These individuals affect the interpersonal aspect of the operation. In particular, the health care providers cannot equate the patient with the pathology that is generating this need for surgery; instead, they must view the patient as a person with whom the doctor, nurses, and the like must interact. A third level at which surgery must be experienced is that which Hackett and Weisman referred to as the impersonal dimension. This is the effect of the disease itself.

Janis [42] noted that patients who only had moderate preoperative anxiety did much better postoperatively than patients with either little anxiety or significantly increased anxiety (ie, the latter two groups suffered greater psychological morbidity). It has been determined that optimistic but honest preoperative counseling with emphasis on the potential benefits is important. In addition, patients do better if given specific activities that will help in the postoperative phase in dealing with pain. It has also been found that undue delays in having the surgery performed significantly increase anticipation and increase the level of stress. However, women seem to need a certain amount of time to come to grips with the prospect of surgery and to prepare themselves emotionally. Women having a hsyterectomy at short notice experienced significantly more depression than women who had a few weeks to process the information.

Menzer et al[43] identified several factors that seem to predict whether or not a woman will present management problems for the nursing staff after a hysterectomy. Women who have a high emotional investment in maintaining their fertility and whose lives revolve around family and motherhood seemed to be at higher risk. The patient's previous history of coping with losses and disappointments in her life also was an important factor. Women who had a pattern of coping with loss by being flexible enough to substitute other satisfactions seemed to recover faster than women who were very rigid and held onto their loss. Patients with a past history of serious or recent losses also were at risk. These findings were replicated by Kaltreider et al,[44] and may partly explain the consistent reports that past history of depression tends to be a complicating factor in recovery.[27,32]

Patients who have a history of coping well with stressful situations have a smoother postoperative course. They admit their anxiety about the surgery to themselves and successfully deal with their fears. Patients who show the most behavior problems postoperatively appear to have few resources to deal with their anxiety. They react with helplessness, panic, impulsivity, and exorbitant demands, much to the chagrin of the nursing staff.

Women who are very invested in their reproductive functions, who have a recent history of significant losses, and who are unable to use their intellect to cope with the anxiety of surgery need a great deal of emotional support. Menzer et al[43] noted that the preoperative psychiatric interview, conducted for the purpose of research, actually seemed to be helpful to the patients in the study; it gave them a chance to establish a relationship with a supportive person prior to surgery, and to verbalize their fears. Coppen et al[45] also noted that the emotional support provided by the researchers in preoperative interviews may have decreased the psychiatric morbidity in their cohorts. Unfortunately, many women go to surgery without the opportunity for a supportive personal talk with their physician, a mental health professional, or a designated liaison nurse.

Sexual Dysfunction

The incidence of sexual dysfunction after hysterectomy has been reported in several series, ranging from 10% to 38%. Unfortunately, as with all summary statements regarding sexual dysfunction, there is no standardization of terms or criteria for diagnosis. The trend, however, appears to suggest a greater incidence with more recent reports. It is unclear whether this is a result of a true change in incidence or a greater sensitivity and acceptance of sexual concerns after hysterectomy. Because these series were gathered as early as 1950 to as recently as 1977, and were collected from different countries, both temporal and cultural variations must be considered.

Masters and Johnson[46] proposed that the three main causes of dyspareunia following hysterectomy were psychological, hormonal, and organic. All have been identified to varying extents in various studies. In an individual case, all these should at least be considered.

There are no consistent data concerning loss of libido or dyspareunia following hysterectomy. Richards[25] reported that some patients experience increased libido because they no longer need to fear conception, whereas others lose some or all sexual desire. Huffman[47] reported that only 10% of women complained of diminished sexual functioning. In contrast, Richards[24] found that 38% of patients, in a general practice survey, felt they had reduced sexual functioning. Martin et al[10] found very small changes in sexual functioning: 32% of the women they studied reported sexual indifference (versus 31% before surgery), 36% (versus 39%) could not achieve a climax, and 27% (versus 22%) complained of dyspareunia. None of these changes were statistically significant. Gath et al[37] reported that 80% of their patients reported return to their preoperative sexual activity by the fourth month after surgery. There also was a significant increase in frequency of intercourse in 56% of patients, and reported enjoyment rose in 39% of cases.

With regard to sexual functioning after hysterectomy, Humphries[48] found that most patients do not have a change in their sexual practices. Feelings of sexual desire, desirability, and sense of femininity were not adversely affected. These findings were contrary to the earlier, less well structured studies in the literature. Because patients in this study received what they considered to be adequate informed consent, a positive outcome may have been due to this factor. In a previous study, Jackson[49] reported that a pamphlet that explained both the operation and the convalescent period improved sexual adjustment and general levels of satisfaction following hysterectomy.

Dennerstein et al,[50] in a retrospective study, found that 36% of patients complained of a deterioration of their sexual relationships that they attributed to the surgery. However, another 34% reported *improved* sexual function, and 29% stated there was no change. The study consisted of interview data from 89 Australian women who had undergone abdominal hysterectomy and bilateral oophorectomy, for reasons other than cancer. Although the study may suffer from not being prospective, the sample was clearly defined and quite homogeneous. The interview was semistructured, lasted about 1 hour, and covered a wide array of relevant topics. Specific questions were asked about changes in desire for sex, enjoyment of sex, vaginal lubrication, ability to reach orgasm, and painful sexual intercourse. The investigators also asked specifically about difficulties in the partner's sexual performance. The interviews took place between 6 months and 5 years after the surgery. The average interval was about 2 years since the operation. Replacement estrogens were taken continuously by 71% of the women and sporadically by 17%; the remaining 12% had not been prescribed estrogens. Significantly more dyspareunia was found in patients who took estrogens sporadically or not at all. However, there was no significant relationship between administration of hormones and desire for sex, enjoyment of sex, ability to reach orgasm, and ease of vaginal lubrication. The most common preoperative anxiety found by Dennerstein et al[50] was fear of being sexually altered (47%). The second most common fear was weight gain (28%).

The presence of preoperative anxiety concerning possible deterioration of sexual functioning was associated with an overall deterioration of sexual relations. Although these data are retrospective in nature, it seems significant that negative expectations, even if verbalized in retrospect, were associated with poor overall sexual outcome and loss of libido. There is a large body of literature in social psychology about the effectiveness of self-fulfilling prophecies.[51] Cultural lore about the sequelae of hysterectomy includes many negative expectations, often firmly held by patients and rarely shared with the physician. In fact, only 10 of the 89 women in the study by Dennerstein et al[50] reported that they had discussed their sexual anxieties with their doctors.

Many patients are too shy to talk about their fears. Some of the myths surrounding hysterectomy that have come to our attention in our clinical work in a large urban teaching hospital in the American South include the following beliefs: a woman with a hysterectomy will become promiscuous or homosexual; she will lose all sexual desire; her partner can tell that she has no uterus even if she has no scar and sex with her will no longer satisfy him; and a husband of a hysterectomized woman will start running around on her because she is now a "hollow woman." It is extremely rare for a patient to talk about these fears openly. There is much "woman-to-woman" gossip that causes anxiety and doubt in the patient. The general consensus seems to be that there are wide individual differences that play a part in women's sexual functioning after a hysterectomy. As in the case of psychiatric symptoms, the best predictor of problems after surgery seems to be a preexisting sexual or marital dysfunction. Although surgical intervention in the area of the reproductive organs is a very threatening prospect for men as well as for women, there is no hard evidence suggesting that hysterectomy, per se, is likely to cause sexual dysfunction in a woman who has a good personal and sexual adjustment and a stable, supportive partner prior to surgery. Since patients are reluctant to approach their physician with concerns about their sexuality, it is important to provide a candidate for hysterectomy with ample opportunity to ask questions and to verbalize any concerns or problems she may have prior to surgery.

Effects of Gynecologic Procedures

Impact of Sterilization Compared with Hysterectomy

As one considers the potential origins of the negative psychosexual impact of hysterectomy, the importance of the sterilizing effect of the procedure has been suggested as a major potential source of problems. Comparing psychological outcome in patients undergoing hysterectomy with those undergoing tubal ligation, there are clear data showing a lower incidence of adverse psychological outcomes after tubal ligation when compared with hysterectomy. Barglow et al[52] matched groups of patients randomly assigned to either tubal ligation or hysterectomy. In this study, 80% of patients undergoing tubal ligation rather than hysterectomy were found to have good long-term psychological adjustment. Since these were patients who did not have any other gynecologic indications for hysterectomy except for sterilization, the data are of limited value today. In contemporary medicine, hysterectomy for elective sterilization is inappropriate, and hysterectomy should be utilized only when medically necessary to treat a specific condition that warrants removal of the uterus.

In general, three different types of adverse psychological reactions have been described after sterilization: regret, psychiatric disturbance, and psychosexual disturbance. Specifically, well-designed studies performed on a prospective basis, using a large sample size, found that sterilization per se is not followed by a high rate of psychiatric disorder. Those studies that did indicate a high level of psychiatric disorder were significantly flawed by their design. Incidence of regret after sterilization has ranged as high as 15%. In general, the percentages usually range from 5 to 10, even though these were women who had been sterilized at their own request. Factors contributing to poststerilization regret included youth and low parity. As in the other two categories, earlier studies indicated higher rates for postoperative sexual dysfunction, with lower rates in more recent, well-designed evaluations.

In general, more recent research indicates that neither sterilization nor hysterectomy results in psychological dysfunction in patients who are otherwise psychiatrically healthy preoperatively. Investigators repeat the caution that interpretation of individual studies must be done in view of different cultural values, different clinical settings, and so forth.

Effect of Oophorectomy

Little has been written in regard to the psychological impact of oophorectomy alone because these investigations have been intermixed with those looking at hysterectomy. This body of literature is very limited, similar to the earlier studies on hysterectomy and sterilization. Of interest, it is the ovaries that produce the female hormones, not the uterus, yet the focus of postoperative psychosocial dysfunction continues to be on the uterus.

Supravaginal Uterine Amputation Versus Total Abdominal Hysterectomy

Another twist on the specific type of hysterectomy was presented by Kilkku et al,[53] who reported on 212 consecutive patients who underwent hysterectomy, 105 of which were total abdominal hysterectomies and 107 of which were supravaginal uterine amputations. Patients were followed for 36 months, with all patients being seen by one interviewer. During the postoperative follow-up period, psychiatric symptoms diminished from those that existed prior to surgery and also from the level at which they were measured 6 weeks after surgery. Of note, there was no increase in depression related to the hysterectomy procedure. The authors interpret the results to "clearly indicate that the view of an increased risk for depression or other psychic complications after hysterectomy should be revised." The percentage of patients without psychiatric symptoms increased from 49.5 preoperatively to 67.7 postoperatively in the hysterectomy group and from 53.3 to 76.8 in the supravaginal uterine amputation group. Both of these were statistically significant. It was also noted that, at 3 years, both nervousness and depression decreased during the follow-up period for the patients undergoing supravaginal uterine amputation but not in the hysterectomy group. The authors suggest that supravaginal uterine amputation may have advantages over total abdominal hysterectomy with regard to psychiatric symptoms.

Dyspareunia after Hysterectomy

Although painful intercourse after hysterectomy is reported by patients, no systematic study has been performed to isolate the effect of performing the hysterectomy from complications of the operation. For example, retained ovaries after the hysterectomy can become involved with adhesions at the vaginal apex, resulting in dyspareunia. Similarly, surgical castration can lead to vaginal atrophy with resultant dyspareunia. Therefore, patients who complain of dyspareunia after hysterectomy must be thoroughly evaluated for both organic as well as psychosexual etiologies. Although a discussion of the issue is not in the scope of this chapter, the operating surgeon must critically assess his or her intraoperative technique with these issues in mind in order to minimize the risk that dyspareunia will occur after hysterectomy.

Just as removal of pelvic pathology causing preoperative dyspareunia can bring great relief to the patient and her partner, postoperative dyspareunia, particularly if there was no problem with preoperative painful intercourse, can be extremely disappointing and must be dealt with in a systematic and forthright fashion. Denial of a potential problem by the physician, with superficial reassurances such as "it will all be fine, just give it time," does not address the total needs of the patient.

Summary

Despite anecdotal reports and extensive media attention, it does not appear from the literature that uncomplicated hysterectomy *per se* directly causes psychologic or sexual problems in patients who did not have significant problems prior to surgery. The questions raised about whether hysterectomy causes these problems do shed important light on the very real problems seen after hysterectomy. Since hysterectomy rarely is an emergency procedure, there usually is time to get to know a patient and to inquire about her personal life, and about what she has heard from other women about the sequelae of hysterectomy. The patient should be questioned regarding her expectations after surgery. Similarly, the operating surgeon should frankly discuss the more common potential complications as well as his or her expectations after surgery. Should there be a significant disparity between patient and physician expectations, further clarification from both may be needed. Once trust and rapport are established, issues such as a history of sexual assault, previous psychiatric problems, marital problems, sexual dysfunction, or negative and fearful anticipations about hysterectomy can be shared prior to surgery. Open communication can pave the way to a potential referral for counseling and support even prior to surgery, thus decreasing the risk for adverse psychological reactions. A realistic preoperative approach by both physician and patient can aid in accurate assessment and management of postoperative problems should they arise.

References

1. Massler DJ, Devansan MM: *Sexual Consequences of Gynecologic Operations in Sexual Consequences of Disability*. Philadelphia, George F. Stickley, 1978.
2. Vieth I: *Hysteria: the History of a Disease*. Chicago, University of Chicago Press, 1965.
3. Guze SB: The role of follow-up studies: Their contribution to diagnostic classification as applied to hysteria. *Semin Psychiatry* 1970;2:392–402.
4. Talbott JA, Hales RE, Yudofsky SC (eds): *Textbook of Psychiatry*. Washington, DC, The American Psychiatric Press, 1988.
5. *Diagnostic and Statistical Manual of Mental Disorders*, ed 3, rev. Washington, DC, American Psychiatric Association, 1987.
6. Ballinger CB: Psychiatric morbidity and the menopause: Survey of a gynecological outpatient clinic. *Br J Psychiatry* 1977;131:83–89.
7. Barker MG: Psychiatric illness after hysterectomy. *BMJ* 1968;2:91–95.
8. Martin RL, Roberts WV, Clayton PJ, et al: Psychiatric illness and non-cancer hysterectomy. *Dis Nerv Syst* 1977;38:974–980.
9. Essen-Möller E, Hagnell O: The frequency and risk of depression within a rural population group in Scania. *Acta Psychiatr Scand* 1961;37(supple 162): 18–32.
10. Martin RL, Roberts WV, Clayton PJ: Psychiatric status after hysterectomy: A one year prospective follow-up. *JAMA* 1980;244:350–353.
11. Perley M, Guze SB: Hysteria: The stability and usefulness of clinical criteria. *N Engl J Med* 1962;266:421–426.
12. Rosenthal TL, Miller ST, Rosenthal RH, et al: Assessing emotional distress at the internist's office. *Behav Res Ther* 1991;29:249–252.
13. Rosenthal TL, Wruble LD, Rosenthal RH, et al: Complaint patterns of patients with irritable bowel syndrome, Crohn's disease and acute gastroenterological illness. *Behav Res Ther* 1987;25:99–112.
14. Waldemar G, Werdelin L, Boysen G: Neurologic symptoms and hysterectomy: A retrospective survey of the prevalence of hysterectomy in neurologic patients. *Obstet Gynecol* 1987;70(4):559–563.
15. Bang J, Dragsted V, Halse C, et al: Hysterectomy: A prospective psychiatric and gynecologic investigation. *Ugeskr Laeger* 1981;143:3035–3040.
16. Dennerstein L, Van Hall EV: *Psychosomatic Gynecology*. Park Ridge, NJ, Parthenon Publishing, 1986, pp 124, 130.
17. Sifneos PE: The prevalence of "alexithymic" characteristics in psychosomatic patients. *Psychother Psychosom* 1973;22:255–262.
18. Shapiro EG, Rosenfeld AA: *The Somatizing Child*. New York, Springer-Verlag, 1986.

19. Lipowski ZJ: Somatization: The concept and its clinical application. *Am J Psychiatry* 1988;145:1358–1368.
20. Ford CV: The somatizing disorders. *Psychosomatics* 1986;27:327–337.
21. Hollender MH: A study of patients admitted to a psychiatric hospital after pelvic operations. *Am J Obstet Gynecol* 1960:79:498–503.
22. Drellich MG, Bieber I: The psychological importance of the uterus and its function. *J Nerv Ment Dis* 1958;126:322–336.
23. Lindemann E: Observations on psychiatric sequelae to surgical operations in women. *Am J Psychiatry* 1941;98:132–137.
24. Richards DH: Depression after hysterectomy. *Lancet* 1973;2:430–432.
25. Richards DH: A post-hysterectomy syndrome. *Lancet* 1974;2:983–985.
26. Bragg RL: Risk of admission to mental hospital following hysterectomy or cholecystectomy. *Am J Public Health* 1965;55:1403–1410.
27. Moore JT, Tolley DH: Depression following hysterectomy. *Psychosomatics* 1976;17:86–89.
28. Meikle S, Brody H: An investigation into the psychological effects of hysterectomy. *J Nerve Ment Dis* 1977;164:36–41.
29. McNair DM, Lorr M, Droppelman LF: *Manual for the Profile of Mood States*. San Diego, CA, Educational and Industrial Testing Service, 1971.
30. Hampton PT, Tarnasky WG: Hysterectomy and tubal ligation: A comparison of the psychological aftermath. *Am J Obstet Gynecol* 1974;119:949–952.
31. Gath D, Cooper P, Day A: Hysterectomy and psychiatric disorder, I: Levels of psychiatric morbidity before and after hysterectomy. *Br J Psychiatry* 1982;140:335–342.
32. Lalinec-Michaud J, Engelsmann F, Marino J: Depression after hysterectomy: A comparative study. *Psychosomatics* 1988;29:307–313.
33. Melody GF: Depressive reactions following hysterectomy. *Am J Obstet Gynecol* 1962;83:410–413.
34. Rosenthal TL, Downs JM, Arheart KL, et al: Similarities and differences on five inventories among mood and anxiety disorder patients. *Behav Res Ther* 1991;29:239–247.
35. Drellich MG, Bieber I: The psychological impact of cancer and cancer surgery. VI. Adaptation to hysterectomy. *Cancer* 1956;9:1120–1126.
36. Ackner B: Emotional aspects of hysterectomy. A follow-up study of 50 patients under the age of 40. *Adv Psychosom Med* 1960;1:248–252.
37. Gath D, Cooper P, Bond A, et al: Hysterectomy and psychiatric disorder, II: Demographic, psychiatric and physical factors in relation to psychiatric outcome. *Br J Psychiatry* 1982;140:343–350.
38. Hendricks-Matthews MK: The importance of assessing a woman's history of sexual abuse before hysterectomy. *J Fam Pract* 1991;32:631–632.
39. Lalinec-Michaud J, Engelsmann F: Cultural factors and reaction to hysterectomy. *Soc Psychiatry Psychiatr Epidemiol* 1989;24:165–171.
40. Ryan MM, Dennerstein L, Pepperell R: Psychological aspects of hysterectomy: A prospective study. *Br J Psychiatry* 1989;154:516–522.
41. Hackett TP, Weisman AS: Psychiatric management of operative syndromes. *Psychosom Med* 1960;22:356.
42. Janis IL: *Psychological Stress*. New York, John Wiley & Sons, 1958.
43. Menzer D, Morris T, Gates P, et al: Patterns of emotional recovery from hysterectomy. *Psychosom Med* 1957;19:379–388.

44. Kaltreider NB, Wallace A, Horowitz MJ: A field study of the stress response syndrome. *JAMA* 1979;242:1499–1503.
45. Coppen A, Bishop M, Beard RJ, et al: Hysterectomy, hormones and behavior: A prospective study. *Lancet* 1981;1:126–128.
46. Masters WH, Johnson VE: *Human Sexual Inadequacy*. Boston, Little, Brown, and Company, 1970, pp 286–287.
47. Huffman JW: The effect of gynecologic surgery on sexual relations. *Am J Obstet Gynecol* 1950;59:915–917.
48. Humphries P: Sexual adjustment after hysterectomy. *Issues in Health Care of Women* 1980;2(2):1–14.
49. Jackson P: Sexual adjustment to hysterectomy and benefits of a pamphlet for patients. *N Z Med J* 1979;90:471–472.
50. Dennerstein L, Wood C, Burrows GD: Sexual response following hysterectomy and oophorectomy. *Obstet Gynecol* 1977;49:92–96.
51. Lindgren HC: *An Introduction to Social Psychology*, ed 2. New York, John Willey & Sons, 1973, pp 227–282.
52. Barglow P, Gunther MS, Johnson A, et al: Hysterectomy and tubal ligation: A psychiatric comparison. *Obstet Gynecol* 1965;25:91–95.
53. Kilkku P, Lehtinen V, Hirvonen T, et al: Abdominal hysterectomy versus supravaginal uterine amputation: Psychic factors. *Ann Chir Gynaecol* 1987; 76(suppl 202):62–67.

Chapter **12**

Residual Ovarian Disease After Hysterectomy

Raymond A. Lee, MD

Anytime a patient undergoes total abdominal hysterectomy and bilateral salpingo-oophorectomy (whether for diffuse endometriosis, pelvic inflammatory disease, or repeat operation after multiple previous pelvic procedures), a small fragment of ovarian tissue may be fixed deep in the pelvic sidewall, or cul-de-sac, or it may be attached to the adjacent bowel and not be removed with the original specimen. Given this situation in a young patient with normal pituitary function and intact pelvic blood supply, the remaining fragment of ovary may continue to function, thus producing ovarian hormones and potentially causing pelvic pain, with or without cyst formation. Surgical and pathologic investigations confirm the presence of ovarian tissue where in fact none would be expected. This situation contrasts with the residual ovarian syndrome in which the ovary is purposely saved, and a pathologic process subsequently develops. Recent data suggest that there is an increase in the incidence of ovarian remnant syndrome. It is more likely that this apparent increase in frequency merely represents the result of more widespread use of ultrasonographic or computerized tomography (CT) scanning in evaluating patients with recurrent or persistent pain after bilateral oophorectomy, thus clarifying the diagnosis.

Incidence

In 1970, Shemwell and Weed[1] described 10 cases of ovarian remnant syndrome and, in 1979, Berek et al[2] emphasized avoiding ureteral damage for this condition and added two additional cases. As a result of increased awareness, an initial study from our institution by Symmonds and Pettit[3] in 1979 reported eight cases, and an additional 31 cases were reported by Pettit and Lee[4] in 1988. In 1991, we saw 19 patients with the ovarian remnant syndrome.

Etiology

Most patients present after having undergone a hysterectomy with bilateral salpingo-oophorectomy for adhesive conditions such as diffuse pelvic endometriosis, pelvic inflammatory disease, or multiple adhesions after previous operations. Because of the loss of normal tissue planes, it may be impossible for the surgeon to recognize and remove all ovarian tissue. All of these patients are premenopausal, and residual fragments of ovary are responsive to stimulation from the pituitary gland and continue to function. Shemwell and Weed[1] demonstrated that fractions of ovarian cortex implanted in cats will continue to function. Two cats exhibited functional ovarian tissue by undergoing estrus. In two other cats, the ovarian cortex became cystic and showed follicular activity, much as we see in humans. It is possible that older patients undergoing oophorectomy under similar conditions may retain portions of the ovary, yet remain asymptomatic because of the lack of ovarian activity.

Clinical Presentation

Most patients present with pelvic pain of highly variable quality—chronic or cyclic—with periodic, sharp, stabbing exacerbations. Usually the pain is located in the pelvis or perineum, but location may vary (right or left side), and dyspareunia is a frequent complaint. When asked, most patients will localize their pain to the same area as the location of the mass, but the patient may have a mass on one side and experience pain on the opposite side or have bilateral pelvic pain. The quality of the pain encompasses the entire range from a pressure sensation and a dull aching to a sharp, severe, and stabbing pain. Some patients may have associated gastrointestinal symptoms, whereas other note urinary tract symptoms. Occasionally, the patients present with a history of having initially experienced hot flashes after their hysterectomy and bilateral salpingo-oophorectomy, only to have these symptoms spontaneously subside after several months, suggesting the renewed function of the remnant of ovary. Occasionally, the cessation of hot flashes coincides with the onset of pelvic discomfort, suggesting the output of estrogen synchronous with the development of pathologic ovarian features. On pelvic examination, a tender, palpable mass or thickening may be noted and the patient's symptoms are reproduced when the mass is palpated. Occasionally, a palpable mass is not found on pelvic examination but will be demonstrated on ancillary tests.

Ancillary Tests

Ultrasonography of the pelvis has been the most effective investigative procedure to define an ovarian remnant. Not infrequently, a nonpalpable mass will be identified by ultrasound; however, there may be an ovarian

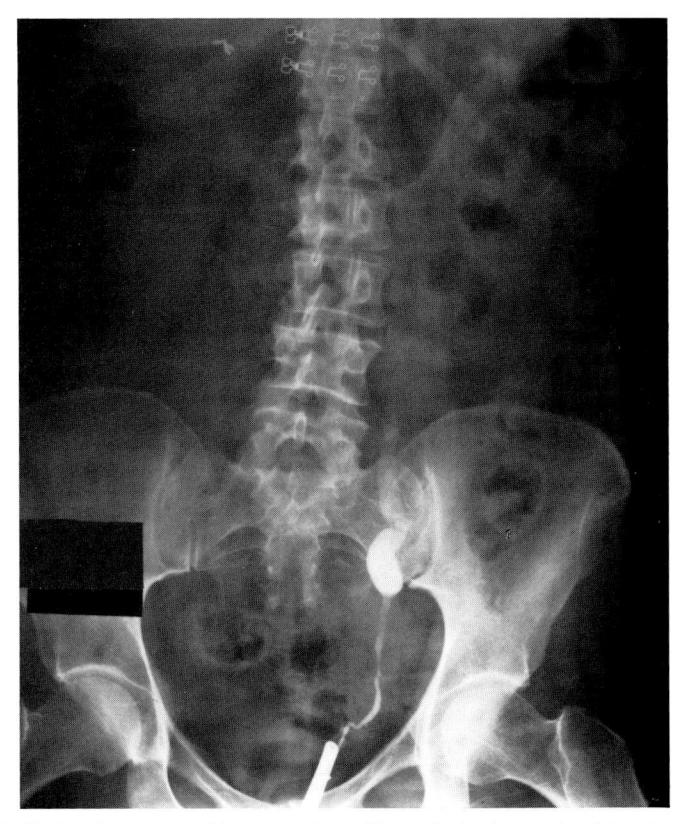

Figure 12.1 Obstructing area of lower ureter with pyelectasis proximal to obstruction. Reprinted, by permission of the American College of Obstetricians and Gynecologists, from Pettit PD, Lee RA: Ovarian remnant syndrome: Diagnostic dilemma and surgical challenge. Obstet Gynecol 1988;71:580–583.

remnant present that is not seen on the ultrasonogram. Computerized tomography has been less effective in our hands for demonstrating an ovarian remnant. Intravenous pyelography may show ureteral dilation or deviation (Figure 12.1). The barium enema may show some extrinsic compression but is usually of little help in making the diagnosis.

We perform laparoscopic examinations infrequently in these patients because adhesions usually prevent accurate assessment of the mass, or the subtle changes may be interpreted as normal without any evidence of the mass. Some investigators have suggested the use of clomiphene citrate to stimulate and enlarge the ovarian remnant to enhance its localization by ultrasound and facilitate its surgical excision.[5]

Follicle-stimulating hormone (FSH) values lend support to the diagnosis. The presence of premenopausal FSH levels in the absence of exogenous hormones confirms that functioning residual ovarian tissue is present. However, patients may have "normal ovarian tissue" excised at operation and yet have had postmenopausal gonadotropin levels preoperatively. This occurrence suggests that the remaining ovarian tissue may not be functioning sufficiently to suppress these hormones. The variable effect of replacement sex steroids on FSH production may complicate the diagnosis and treatment of the ovarian remnant syndrome.

Treatment

Nonoperative Management

Cyclic estrogen and progesterone therapy may be acceptable nonoperative alternatives.[6] The use of danazol has resulted in symptom reduction, but we have not found this to yield effective long-term management of the problem. Radiotherapy has been reported[1] to be successful in some patients given castrating levels of radiation. We have encountered patients who have received 10 Gy before being seen at our institution, with no beneficial effect on their symptoms and persistence of the pelvic mass.

Before being seen at our institution, approximately 50% of the patients have undergone previous operations (1 to 7), specifically for excision of the ovarian remnant.

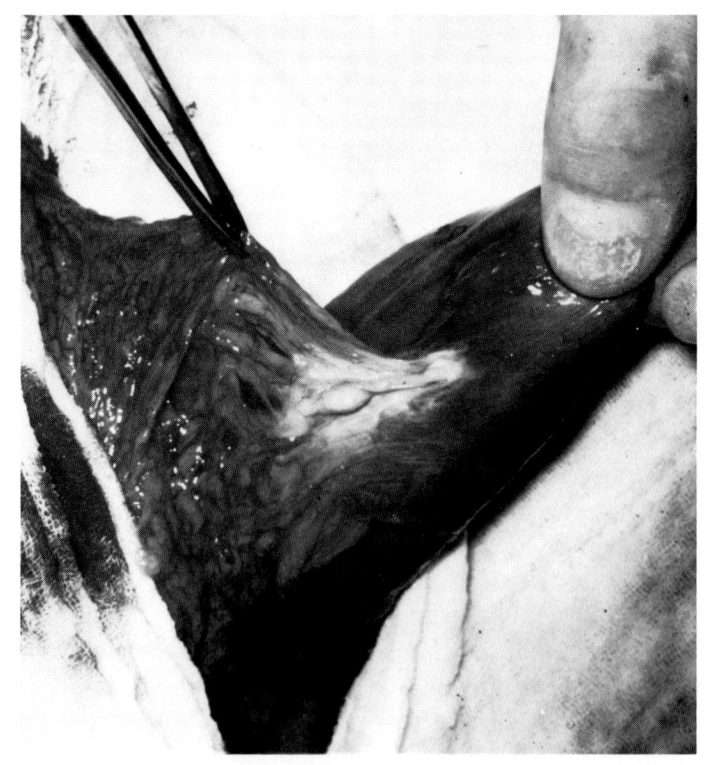

Figure 12.2 Islet of ovarian remnant on mesentary of ileum and omentum. *Reprinted, by permission of the American College of Obstetricians and Gynecologists, from Symmonds RE, Pettit PDM: Ovarian remnant syndrome. Obstet Gynecol 1979;54:174–177.*

Operative Procedures

A thorough abdominal and pelvic exploration (preferably through a large, lower abdominal incision), including examination of the small and large intestines, is necessary. The ovarian remnant may present as a parasitic attachment to the intestine (Figure 12.2) without any evidence of disease within the pelvis. The operative dissection is begun by clamping and cutting the round ligament, opening the broad ligament with the development of the perirectal and perivesical spaces, and dividing the anterior division of the internal iliac vessels. This "sets up" the operative approach to facilitate the dissection of the ureter.

We favor beginning the retroperineal dissection of the ureter above the level of the previous operation. Berek et al[2] advocated preoperative placement of a ureteral stent to safeguard against ureteral injury. Our experience suggests that the presence of the ureteral stent might prove helpful in those patients with multiple previous operative procedures. However, because of its firm nature, a stent potentially could add to the risk of ureteral injury. If significant ureteral trauma is anticipated or if a ureteral stent would be helpful in delineating the ureter, an extraperitoneal retropubic cystotomy may be performed and a ureteral catheter passed retrograde (Figure 12.3). When mobilizing the ureter, the surgeon should stay close to the ureter and apply tension to the mass to provide

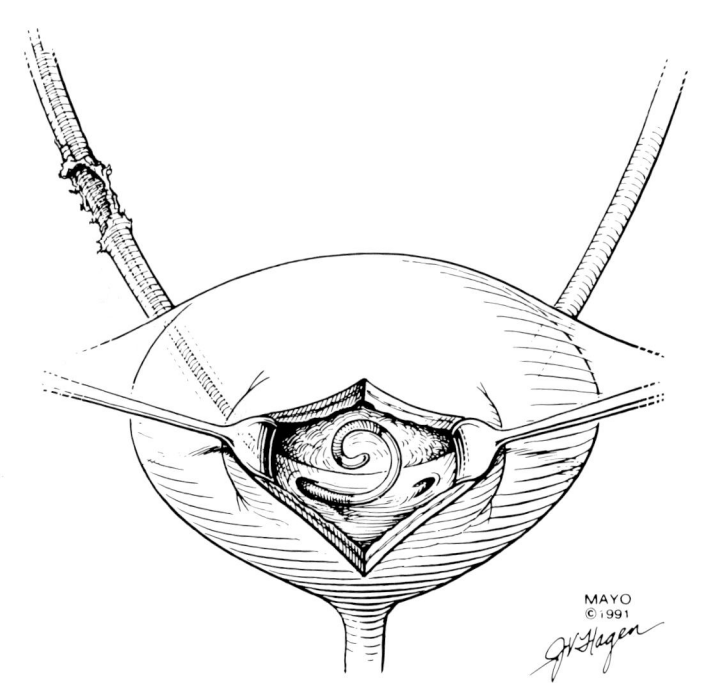

Figure 12.3 Through the cystotomy, the ureteral catheter is passed up the ureter in a retrograde fashion. *Reprinted, by permission of Mayo Foundation, from Lee RA: Urinary tract, in Lee RA (ed): Atlas of Gynecologic Surgery, Philadelphia, WB Saunders, 1992, p 303.*

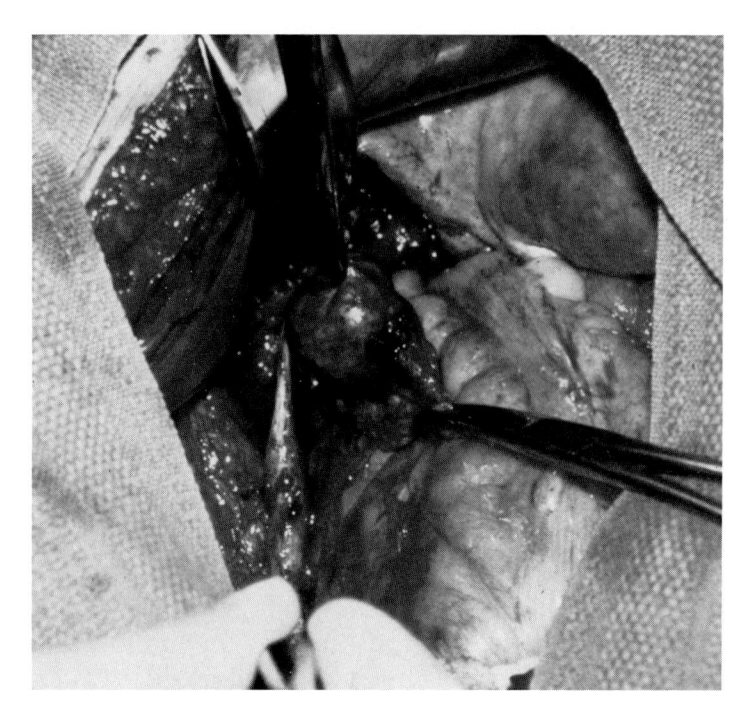

Figure 12.4 Cystic ovarian remnant under tension, with narrowed ureter being compressed on its lateral surface. *Reprinted, by permission of the American College of Obstetricians and Gynecologists, from Pettit PD, Lee RA: Ovarian remnant syndrome: Diagnostic dilemma and surgical challenge. Obstet Gynecol 1988;71:580–583.*

necessary countertraction for sharp dissection (Figure 12.4). Rather than concentrating on excision of the mass, attention is directed to complete dissection of the ureter throughout its pelvic course (Figure 12.5). After this is accomplished, my colleagues and I completely excise the ovarian remnant with its contiguous peritoneum and surrounding tissues. We also do the same exploration on the opposite side, despite the lack of symptoms. This is done to ensure that there is no "silent" remnant present that could lead to symptoms and repeat operation at a later date. In most patients and in all those undergoing repeat operation, Hemovac catheter drainage is done in an extraperitoneal fashion to prevent hematoma or lymphocyst formation.

Operative Findings

In about half the specimens, a corpus luteum is found. One third of our patients had normal ovarian tissue, and about one quarter had ovarian endometriosis. Other findings included follicular cysts and benign ovarian tumors such as ovarian fibroma, serous cystadenoma, and papillary serous cystadenoma.

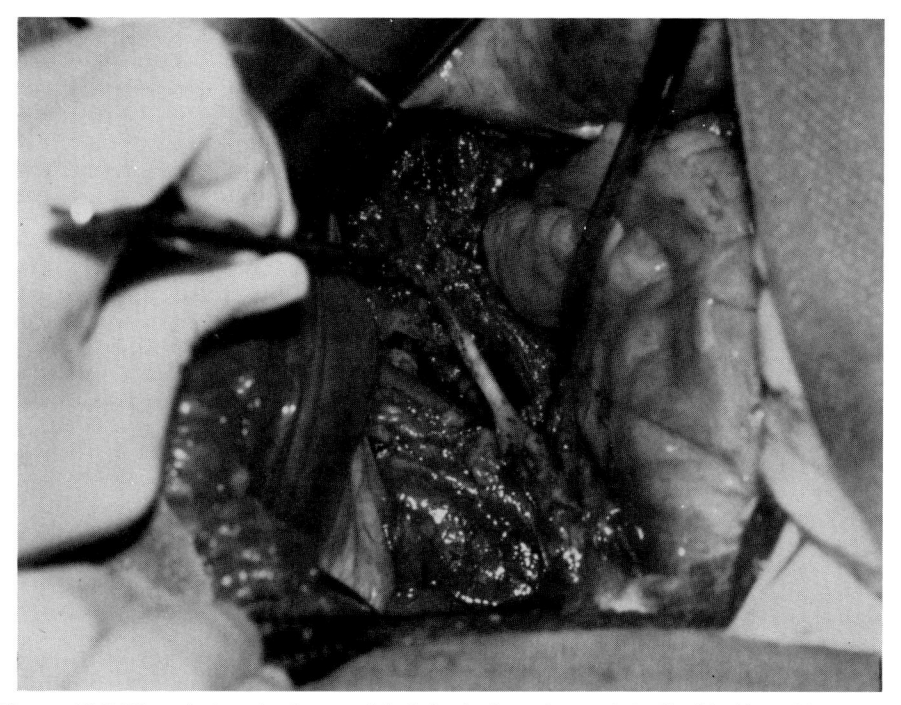

Figure 12.5 Dissected ureter from pelvic brim to its entrance into the bladder with narrow, cordlike ureter intact. Repeat intravenous pyelography 2 months after operation showed normal function with no evidence of narrowing or obstruction of the left ureter. *Reprinted, by permission of the American College of Obstetricians and Gynecologists, from Pettit PD, Lee RA: Ovarian remnant syndrome: Diagnostic dilemma and surgical challenge. Obstet Gynecol 1988;71:580–583.*

Complications

The overwhelming majority of our patients experience prompt relief of symptoms and an uncomplicated postoperative course. Rarely will the patient require transfusion; infrequently, a portion of the colon or small bowel will be removed en bloc with the specimen to ensure complete excision. Significant postoperative ileus was uncommon, and no patients experienced gastrointestinal or gastrourinary fistula. Those patients with endometriosis are treated with progestational agents for 3 to 6 months before reinitiating estrogen-replacement therapy.

Summary

The patient with ovarian remnant syndrome, an unusual complication of bilateral oophorectomy, usually presents with pelvic pain with or without a mass. Various adhesion-producing conditions leading to retention of ovarian tissue—such as endometriosis, pelvic inflammatory disease, or inflammatory bowel disease—were present at the original procedure.

The relative increase in diagnosis of this condition during the past 5 years may represent a greater awareness of the potential condition, combined with a wider use of ultrasonography and CT scanning. Surgical correction requires dissection and mobilization of the ureter throughout its entire pelvic course to facilitate resection of the specimen. The complications are minor, and symptoms will be relieved.

References

1. Shemwell RE, Weed JC: Ovarian remnant syndrome. *Obstet Gynecol* 1970;36:299–303.
2. Berek JS, Darney PD, Lopkin C, et al: Avoiding ureteral damage in pelvic surgery for ovarian remnant syndrome. *Am J Obstet Gynecol* 1979;133:221–222.
3. Symmonds RE, Pettit PDM: Ovarian remnant syndrome. *Obstet Gynecol* 1979;54:174–177.
4. Pettit PD, Lee RA: Ovarian remnant syndrome: Diagnostic dilemma and surgical challenge. *Obstet Gynecol* 1988;71:580–583.
5. Kaminski PF, Sorosky JI, Mandell MJ, et al: Clomiphene citrate stimulation as an adjunct in locating ovarian tissue in ovarian remnant syndrome. *Obstet Gynecol* 1990;76:924–926.
6. Nelson DC, Avant GR: Ovarian remnant syndrome. *South Med J* 1982;75:757–758.

Chapter **13**

Laparoscopic-Assisted Vaginal Hysterectomy

Thomas G. Stovall, MD, and Robert L. Summitt, Jr, MD

Hysterectomy is second only to cesarean section as the most frequently performed surgical procedure in the United States. Of the total number of hysterectomies performed, approximately 25% to 30% are done vaginally. Berengarius of Bologna is thought to be the first surgeon to have documented removal of the uterus through the vagina. Other sources credit Andreas of Cruce for performing the first vaginal hysterectomy in 1560. However, prior to this time Soranus, a Greek obstetrician of Alexandria and Aretaeus, and Paulus Aeginata referred to the idea of vaginal hysterectomy in their writings.[1]

As described by Chatman and Cohen,[2] Kelling,[3,4] in 1902 using a model, is given credit as the first person to perform celioscopy, and Jacobaeus[5] was the first person to perform laparoscopy in the human. Because of the ability to perform minimally invasive surgery, especially on an outpatient basis, the use of diagnostic and operative laparoscopy has increased dramatically over the last 10 years.

History and Results of Laparoscopy with Hysterectomy

Laparoscopic-assisted vaginal hysterectomy has been introduced as an alternative surgical approach to standard methods of abdominal and vaginal hysterectomy. The first reported case of laparoscopic-assisted hysterectomy was performed by Reich et al[6] on a patient with pelvic pain secondary to adhesions from previous surgical treatment (laparoscopic salpingo-ovariolysis and laser vaporization of mild endometriosis) and menorrhagia secondary to uterine myomas. The technique described in this report included aquadissection, bipolar electrocautery, and carbon dioxide (CO_2) laser, with a total operative time of 180 minutes. The patient was discharged on the fourth postoperative day and returned to her normal activities within 3 weeks. This initial case report was followed by the report of Nezhat et al,[7] who first utilized the endoscopic titanium multifire

GIA stapling device to ligate the surgical pedicles. In addition, these authors used individual clips on one side, and the CO_2 laser to ligate the uterine artery on the opposite side.

Kovac et al[8] reported the use of diagnostic laparoscopy in 46 patients who had been advised to have an abdominal hysterectomy by their referring gynecologic surgeon. In this study, patients were assigned a numerical laparoscopic score based on uterine size, adnexal mobility, the presence or absence of pelvic adhesions, endometriosis, and cul-de-sac pathology as diagnosed by laparoscopy. In many patients, uterine size was overestimated and uterine mobility was underestimated on the preoperative bimanual examination. It is also of interest that ovarian pathology was suspected in 14 cases at the time of referral, and ultrasound and pelvic examinations confirmed the suspicion in only 8 (47%) patients. All eight of the patients had the diagnosis disproven at the time of laparoscopy. It was also the authors' opinion that the lysis of ovarian adhesions did not increase the utilization of the vaginal approach. Following laparoscopy, 42 of 46 patients (98%) were considered to be candidates and underwent successful vaginal hysterectomy.

Nezhat et al[9] prospectively randomized 20 patients with a uterine size of 14 weeks' gestation equivalent or less who were considered candidates for abdominal hysterectomy. Seven of ten patients in the abdominal hysterectomy group, two of whom had a history of previous surgery, were operated on for leiomyomata. The mean uterine weight was 213 g (range 60 to 534). Although some of these patients had previous stage III-IV endometriosis, no mention was made in the article regarding the status of their endometriosis at the time of hysterectomy. In the ten patients randomized to laparoscopic-assisted hysterectomy, two were operated on for leiomyomata and seven were operated on for stage III-IV endometriosis. Again, the current stage of endometriosis in these patients was not reported. Although not part of this study protocol, these authors reported as an addendum to this study a total of 96 laparoscopic hysterectomies. These cases establish the safety and feasibility of the operative approach when performed by experienced laparoscopic surgeons. However, they did not establish any benefit to this approach over vaginal hysterectomy or abdominal hysterectomy. This can only be determined through rigorously controlled randomized trials.

At the 1991 American Family Society Meeting, Fernandez et al[10] reported 25 cases of laparoscopic-assisted vaginal hysterectomies done for what these investigators believed were contraindications to standard vaginal hysterectomy. Surgical indications in this group included nulliparity (7 cases), previous pelvic laparotomy (9), organic ovarian cysts (4), pelvic endometriosis/adenomyosis (3), prior sacral fixation (1), and bilateral hydrosalpinx (1). A prophylactic bilateral salpingo-oophorectomy was performed in 15 patients age 50 years or older. The surgical technique used included bipolar electrocoagulation, with a mean operative time of

115 ± 29 minutes (range 85 to 165) and a mean postoperative hospitalization of 4.2 ± 1.7 days (range 3 to 8). The postoperative convalescence period was reported not to exceed 1 month.

Summitt et al[11] reported, the results of a prospective randomized trial that included 56 women scheduled for vaginal hysterectomy. Patients were randomly assigned to undergo either a laparoscopic-assisted vaginal hysterectomy with endoscopic staples ($n = 29$) or a standard vaginal hysterectomy ($n = 27$). The most common indication in this group of patients was leiomyomata uteri, and the second most common indication was pelvic pain of uterine origin unresponsive to conservative therapy. The mean operative time in the laparoscopic-assisted group (120.1 ± 28.5 minutes) was approximately twice that of the standard vaginal hysterectomy group (64.7 ± 27.0 minutes). There was no statistical difference in the mean uterine weight between the laparoscopic-assisted group and the standard vaginal hysterectomy group (162.6 ± 89.5 versus 203.7 ± 143.0 g, respectively). The estimated blood loss in the laparoscopic-assisted group (203.8 ± 130.5 mL) was statistically less than that in the standard hysterectomy group (376.1 ± 261.5 mL). However, the postoperative hematocrits were statistically higher in the vaginal hysterectomy group when compared to the laparoscopic-assisted group. Oophorectomies were successfully completed in all cases in which they were indicated. All procedures were performed on an outpatient basis, with the mean hospital cost being $4,891 ± $355 (range $4,311 to $5,247) for vaginal hysterectomy and $7,905 ± $501 (range $7,197 to $8,289) for laparoscopic-associated vaginal hysterectomy. Postoperative pain and antiemetic medication required were the same in both groups, except on postoperative day 2, in which patients undergoing laparoscopic-assisted vaginal hysterectomy required significantly more pain medication than patients undergoing standard hysterectomy.

Liu reviewed his experience with 72 women who underwent laparoscopic hysterectomy using a combination of bipolar electrocoagulation, CO_2 laser, and operative laparoscopy.[12] No complications were reported in this series. Indications for surgery included adenomyosis, pelvic pain with proven or suspected endometrium, adhesive disease, and leiomyoma. Twenty-nine patients had undergone previous pelvic surgery. Concomitant surgical procedures included salpingo-oophorectomy ($n = 49$), vaporization and/or excision of endometriosis implants ($n = 26$), adhesiolysis ($n = 45$), and appendectomy ($n = 14$). Liu reported an average hospitalization cost of $3,772.00. This report confirms the feasibility of performing the procedure, but without specific controls and a comparison group no further conclusions can be drawn. Other statements made in the discussion of this paper, such as less discomfort when compared with abdominal hysterectomy as a result of tissue desiccation rather than suturing, decreased adhesion formation, and decreased pulmonary problems, cannot be substantiated. Again, these issues can only be resolved in prospective, randomized trials.

Operative Technique Using Multifire Endoscopic Staples

Laparoscopic-assisted vaginal hysterectomy was initially accompanied by long operating times, expensive equipment, and the need for increased surgical skill. The introduction of endoscopic multifire titanium staples has reduced operating times and potentially improved on the safety of the procedure by obviating the need for bipolar cautery. Since laparoscopic and vaginal surgery techniques are combined, necessary instrumentation is obtained from both standard laparoscopic (or pelviscopic) equipment and standard vaginal surgery equipment (Table 13.1).

Following induction of general anesthesia, the patient is placed in the dorsal lithotomy position. Although several types of stirrups can be used, we prefer the "candy-cane" stirrups because they allow adequate exposure during both the vaginal and laparoscopic portions of the surgical procedure. Setting the stirrups at their lowest adjustment point keeps the thighs out of the operative field during the laparoscopic portion of the operation.

Following an examination under anesthesia, the perineum, vagina, and lower abdomen are prepped with a dilute povidone-iodine solution. A Hulka tenaculum is attached to the cervix through a side-opening Graves speculum, making certain to antevert the uterus. A Foley catheter is inserted and the patient is draped using standard laparoscopy drapes. A 12-mm trocar is inserted periumbilically. Following correct placement

Table 13.1 Instrumention Needed to Perform a Laparoscopic-Assisted Vaginal Hysterectomy with Endoscopic Staples

Pelviscopic surgical equipment
A 10-mm, 0° telescope
A 45°-angled-lens telescope
Three 12-mm trocars and sleeves
A 5-mm grasping forceps (traumatic/atraumatic)
Two 5.5- or 4.5-mm operating port convertors
One 10.5-mm operating port convertor
Hook-scissors with electrocautery capability
Unipolar/bipolar cautery
Suction/irrigation system
Hulka tenaculum
Endoscopic surgical stapler
Vaginal hysterectomy equipment
"Candy-cane" stirrups

and gas insufflation of the abdomen, two 12-mm trocars are placed in the right and left lower quadrants, 6 to 8 cm above the pubic rami and lateral to the inferior epigastric vessels. The placement of three 12-mm trocars allows for maximum flexibility of insertion and direction of the endoscopic stapling device. With all three trocar sheaths in place, a full abdominal survey is performed, taking particular note of the presence of adhesions and upper abdominal pathology. This survey includes an examination of the uterus, tubes, ovaries, and cul-de-sac.

Once the abdominal and pelvic surveys are complete, the first true step of the operation is to develop and mobilize the bladder flap. Beginning at the left round ligament, the peritoneum of the vesicouterine fold is incised with the hook scissors. Attaching the unipolar cautery to the hook scissors allows for an easier dissection with less blood obscuring the operative field. The incision is continued across the lower uterine segment to the opposite round ligament. On completing the incision, the bladder is sharply dissected off the lower uterine segment and cervix. This is best accomplished by lifting the lower peritoneal edge with graspers, and using hook scissors to incise and dissect the loose areolar tissue and bladder from the uterus. To maintain good hemostasis, activate the unipolar cautery prior to cutting. A contact-tip neodymium:yttrium-aluminum-garnet laser may also be used for dissection. Once the bladder flap has been developed, the ureters are identified by incising the medial leaf of the broad ligament and dissecting to retroperitoneal space in a manner similar to that of performing an abdominal hysterectomy.

The proper disposable reloading unit for the Endo-Gauge must be determined before inserting the Endo-GIA. The Endo-Gauge is inserted through the periumbilical port, incorporating the upper pedicle. Once the proper reload is selected and attached to the Endo-GIA, the instrument is inserted through the lower port on the same side of the uterus that is to be stapled. Grasping forceps are inserted through the other opposite lower port. The upper pedicle is visualized while pushing the uterus up and to the opposite side. The Endo-GIA is opened the round ligament, fallopian tube, and uteroovarian ligament are enclosed. This is best performed with the reloading unit directed forward. If the ovaries are to be removed, the device is placed lateral to the ovary, incorporating the infundibulopelvic ligament. The unit must be pushed open fully to the hinge joint and must be adjacent to the uterus. The tip of the stapler should be past the cut edge of anterior peritoneum. Once properly positioned, the stapling unit is closed and locked in place. The closed position is inspected, paying particular attention that no bowel is enclosed and that the ureter is free. The safety is released and the stapling unit is activated. After removing the stapling unit, the cut and stapled edges are inspected for hemostasis and proper staple alignment. If these are satisfactory, the same procedure is performed on the opposite side. Alternatively, the uterine artery of the same side may be staple-ligated next. To staple-ligate the uterine artery, the uterus is again pushed upward and to the opposite side from the one being stapled. The Endo-GIA is opened and aligned vertically along the uterus, incorporating the uterine artery. A white 3.0 V reload is typically used for this step. The open Endo-GIA is pushed down to the apex of the previously cut pedicle, the stapler is closed, and again the position of the ureter is inspected. If satisfactory, the stapler is fired and removed slowly, checking for hemostasis. The procedure is repeated on the opposite side.

In most cases, the endoscopic portion of the surgery is completed after ligation and division of the uterine arteries. The level of the bladder and vagina prevents further downward application of staples. In some cases, however (if the bladder is adequately dissected and displaced), the upper aspect of the cardinal ligaments may be staple-ligated, using the same principles demonstrated earlier. It is extremely important to visualize and avoid the ureter during this step. Although not mandatory, we routinely enter the vagina through an anterior colpotomy incision during the laparoscopic portion of this operation. Posterior cul-de-sac entry has also been used, but we do not routinely perform this step.

When the endoscopic dissection is complete, the vaginal approach is begun. Adequate exposure is obtained and the Hulka tenaculum removed. A tenaculum is applied to the cervix and the vaginal hysterectomy is begun in a standard fashion through a posterior cul-de-sac entry. After entering the posterior cul-de-sac, the uterosacral ligaments are ligated, and a deaver or right-angle retractor is placed in the anterior cul-de-sac. We find it helpful to palpate the next pedicle, feeling the staple line from below, in order to direct clamp placement. Once the final portion of the broad ligament has been clamped, cut, and ligated, the uterus is removed. The vagina is closed in a standard fashion with interrupted delayed absorbable suture.

We routinely reestablish a pneumoperitoneum and inspect for hemostatis with the laparoscope, irrigating the pelvis with saline. The patient may then be taken to the recovery room. In the majority of cases, our patients are discharged home on the same day of surgery.

Role of Laparoscopic Assistance

With these limited available data, what, then, is the role of laparoscopy before or as a part of vaginal hysterectomy? Laparoscopy as a diagnostic procedure, when used as an aid to determine the extent of intraabdominal pathology, has been shown by Kovac et al[8] to increase the number of patients who were candidates for a vaginal approach to hysterectomy. However, is this really practical? If one adds laparoscopy to a large number of patients prior to hysterectomy, one loses or diminishes several of the advantages of vaginal hysterectomy, particularly decreased operative/anesthesia time. Also, one adds cost to the procedure and adds the risk and morbidity of laparoscopy. If this view is modified to include laparoscopic assessment, only those patients with risk factors for endometriosis or pelvic adhesive disease must be considered. First, not all patients with historic or pelvic examination predictors of adhesions are actually found to have adhesions. Second, even if these predictors are present, this does not necessarily preclude a vaginal approach to hysterectomy. Therefore, laparoscopy prior to vaginal hysterectomy does not appear practical.

In a study published from the University of Tennessee, Memphis,[13] the presence of any of the following historic or physical findings identified the patient as one suspected of having adhesions based on the preoperative assessment: (1) previous treatment for pelvic inflammatory disease, (2) previously documented endometriosis, (3) previous pelvic or abdominal surgery, (4) previously documented pelvic adhesions, (5) previously documented tubal occlusion, (6) a history of chronic pelvic pain of at least 6 months' duration, (7) cervical motion tenderness, (8) uterine tenderness, (9) adnexal tenderness, (10) palpable adnexal mass, and (11) uterine immobility. In this study, 67 patients had at least one historic predictor of adhesions, of whom 35 (52.2%) had adhesive disease, leaving 32 (47.8%) patients who had no adhesions. Thirty patients had two historic predictors of adhesions; 17 (56.7%) of them had adhesions found at laparoscopy. Forty-seven of 176 (26.7%) patients had no historic predictors of adhesions present, and were found not to have adhesions at the time of laparoscopy. It is true that, if the patient had one or more historic predictors of adhesions, she was statistically more likely to have adhesions than if she had no predictors ($p > .05$). However, in almost 50% of patients with a predictor there was no adhesive disease, and in nearly 30% of patients with adhesions there was no historic predictor present. In this study the false-negative rate for a normal physical examination was 32%, and the false-negative rate for patients with both a negative history and normal physical examination was 25.6%.

The use of operative laparoscopic techniques to ligate the infundibulopelvic or uteroovarian ligaments, uterine artery, and cardiac ligament is a proposed technique to increase the utilization of the vaginal approach. Various techniques, advantages, and disadvantages as well as preoperative indications have been proposed. There is no consensus as to the proper circumstances under which operative laparoscopic techniques would be helpful. We do know that, when standard vaginal hysterectomy can be performed, there is no advantage to adding the laparoscopic approach. In fact, the data by Summitt et al[11] show several disadvantages to this approach. To date, there are no data available showing that an intended abdominal hysterectomy can be converted to a vaginal approach. Because the laparoscopic-assisted procedure is new, operator experience is lacking, as are well-defined indications.

In the absence well-defined indications for this technique, proposed reasons for performing laparoscopic-assisted vaginal hysterectomy relate to conditions that might require abdominal surgery or contraindicate a vaginal approach. Some examples of these conditions are: (1) chronic pelvic pain that has not responded to conservative therapy, (2) leiomyomata uteri, (3) endometriosis or a prior history of endometriosis, (4) pelvic adhesive disease, (5) potential benign adnexal pathology, and (6) poor uterine mobility. Currently, there are no data to support the supposition that patients undergoing hysterectomy for pelvic pain or a prior history of endometriosis are not candidates for a vaginal approach. There is no current way to standardize the preoperative assessment of these patients, which must be done before it can be determined if abdominal hysterectomy can be replaced in some instances with a laparoscopic-assisted approach.

Others have noted that, if the ovaries are to be removed (in patients over 40 years of age), the laparoscopic approach offers the advantage of being able to remove the ovaries during vaginal hysterectomy. In our experience, it is very unusual not to be able to remove the ovaries during a standard vaginal approach.[11] In our view, a laparoscopic-assisted approach should not be used by the surgeon who is not already well trained in vaginal surgery.

The addition of laparoscopy does not necessarily simplify the procedure, and in many instances complicates it. In the future, it may be possible to use these techniques on patients with early-stage endometrial or ovarian cancer. The approach in these patients would include laparoscopy with cytology, assisted vaginal hysterectomy, bilateral salpingo-oophorectomy, and lymph node sampling. The first two cases of a laparoscopic-assisted radical hysterectomy with paraaortic and pelvic lymphadenectomy for treatment of a stage $1A_2$ carcinoma of the cervix were recently reported.[14] Techniques used included bipolar electrocoagulation, CO_2 laser, and hydrodissection. The operating times in the two cases were 7 and 6 hours. This is a potentially promising technique. However, larger series with multicenter randomized trials to fairly assess the complications are mandatory.

We have shown that both vaginal hysterectomy and laparoscopic-assisted hysterectomy can be successfully performed on an outpatient basis.[15] At the present time, the addition of laparoscopic instrumentation and sampling devices has broadened our gynecologic surgical horizons. Reporting of small case series without well-established criteria only proves that the operation can be safely accomplished. Randomized prospective trials can and must be done before the advantages, disadvantages, and complications of this technology can be elucidated.

References

1. Benrubi GI: History of hysterectomy. *J Fla Med Assoc* 1988;75:533–538.
2. Chatman DL, Cohen MR: History of endoscopy, in Martin DC, Holz GL, Levinson CJ, et al (eds): *Manual of Endoscopy*. Santa Fe Springs, CA, The American Association of Gynecologic Laparoscopists, 1990, pp 1–10.

3. Kelling G: Uber Oesophagos Kopie, Gastroskopie and Kolioskopie. *Med Wochenschr (Munich)* 1902;49:21–25.
4. Nitze M: Uber eine neue Beleuch turgsmethope der Hchlen des Menschilchen Korpens. *Wein Med Presse* 1879;26:87–92
5. Jocobaeus HC: Uber die Moglichkeit die Zystokope be: Untersuchung Seroser Hohluns Anzuwenden. *Med Wochenschr (Munich)* 1910;57:2070–2074.
6. Reich H, De Caprio J, McGlynn F: Laparoscopic-hysterectomy. *J Gynecol Surg* 1989;5:213–216.
7. Nezhat C, Nezhat F, Silfen SL: Laparoscopic hysterectomy and bilateral salpingo-oophorectomy using multifire GIA surgical stapler. *J Gynecol Surg* 1990;6:287–288.
8. Kovac SR, Cruikshank SH, Retto WF: Laparoscopy-assisted vaginal hysterectomy. *J Gynecol Surg* 1990;6:185–193.
9. Nezhat F, Nezhat C, Gordon S, et al: Laparoscopic versus abdominal hysterectomy. *J Repro Med* 1992;37:247–250.
10. Fernandez H, Lelaidier C, Frydman R: Laparoscopic approach for vaginal hysterectomy: A new surgical approach. Read at the 47th Annual Meeting of the American Fertility Society, Oct 22, 1991.
11. Summitt RL Jr, Stovall TG, Lipscomb GH, et al: Randomized comparison of laparoscopic-assisted vaginal hysterectomy versus standard vaginal hysterectomy in an outpatient setting. *Obstet Gynecol*, in press.
12. Liu CY: Laparoscopic hysterectomy: A review of 72 cases. *J Reprod Med* 1992;37:351–354.
13. Stovall TG, Elder RE, Ling FW: Predictor of pelvic adhesion. *J Reprod Med* 1989;34:345–348.
14. Nezhat CR, Burrell MO, Nezhat FR, et al: Laparoscopic radical hysterectomy with paraaortic and pelvic node dissection. *Am J Obstet Gynecol* 1992;166:864–865.
15. Stovall TG, Summitt RL Jr, Bran DF, et al: Outpatient vaginal hysterectomy: A pilot study. *Obstet Gynecol*, 1992;80:143–150.

Index

Note: Page numbers followed by f refer to illustrations, page numbers followed by t refer to tables.

A

Abdominal hysterectomy
  indications for, 28–29
  psychiatric aspects of, 177–178
  pulmonary complications, 7
Abdominal tenderness, postoperative, 159
Abdominoplasty, 127
Abnormal bleeding, without obvious cause, 23
Abortion, 23
Abscess
  pelvic, 159–160
  tuboovarian, 142
Actinomyces israelii, 134
Administration route, and antibiotic prophylactic efficacy, 42–43
Adnexal pathology, 23
Adnexectomy, 142
Adrenocortical steroids, postoperative, 152
Alexithymia, 168
Allergic reactions, postoperative, 160
Ambulation, postoperative, 154
Analgesia, patient-controlled, 150
Anaphylaxis, 43
Angiographic arterial embolization, 95–97
Antibiotic therapy
  comparative trials. *See* Antibiotic trials
  distant infection incidence, 42
  financial advantages of, 40, 42
  infection risk factors, 36–37
  in pelvic inflammatory disease, 138–140
  and platelet dysfunction, 82
  prophylactic, 12–13, 35–43, 152
  route of administration and, 42–43
  single-dose prophylaxis, 43
Antibiotic trials, 37–40
  abdominal hysterectomy
    comparative prophylaxis, 41t–42t
    placebo-controlled, 40t
  vaginal hysterectomy
    comparative prophylaxis, 38t-39t
    placebo-controlled, 37t
Anticoagulation therapy, 9
Antiinflammatory medications, and platelet dysfunction, 82
Anxiety, 169–173
Appendectomy, concurrent, 125–126
Arrhythmias, ventricular, 157
Aspirin, and platelet dysfunction, 82
Asthma, bronchial, 7
Atelectasis, 156

B

Babcock clamp, 92f, 93
Barium edema, and ovarian remnant syndrome, 185
Behavior problems, posthysterectomy, 173–174
Bernard-Soulier syndrome, 83
Bethanechol, 151
Biopsy, endometrial, 4
Bivalving, and uterine morcellation, 103
Bladder drainage, postoperative, 150–151
Bladder injuries, 51–59
  fistulas, 52–59
  prevention of, 52
  repair of, 52–53
    closure, 54f
    space of Retzius development, 53f

Bleeding. *See also* Hemorrhage
　acquired disorders, 80–82
　　disseminated intravascular
　　　coagulation, 80–81
　　platelet disorders, 82
　　procoagulant disorders, 82
　　secondary to transfusion, 81–82
　categories of, 79
　congenital disorders, 82–83
　　platelet disorders, 82–83
　　procoagulant disorders, 82
　intraoperative, 83–98
　　anatomy of pelvic bleeding, 84–85
　　angiographic arterial embolization, 95–97
　　assessment of, 83–84
　　hypogastric artery ligation, 89–95
　　infundibulopelvic ligament hematoma, 88
　　initial management of, 84
　　management principles, 87–88
　　military antishock trousers, 97–98
　　pelvic packs, 88–89
　　physiology of pelvic bleeding, 85
　　prevention of, 85–87
　posthysterectomy, 98–99
　preoperative diagnosis of, 83
Blood glucose level, 5
Blood tests, 5
Boari-Ockerblad method, 64f, 65
Bowel cleansing, 11
Bowel injuries, 66–75
　avoiding during abdominal surgery, 68t
　bowel preparations, 67, 67t
　conditions associated with, 67t
　prevention, 67–68
　superficial and minor injury repair, 68–70
　　longitudinal tear, 69f, 69–70
　　small puncture injury, 68f, 68–69
　unrecognized injuries, 70–75
　　diagnosis, 70
　　large bowel injuries, 73–75
　　repair timing, 70
　　small bowel injuries, 70–73, 71f–74f
Briquet's syndrome, 164–169
　clinical approach to, 167–169
　frequency of symptoms in, 167t
Bronchitis, 8

C

Cancer
　as indication for hysterectomy, 22
　ovarian, and oophorectomy, 117–118
Cardiovascular complications, postoperative, 157–158
Cardiovascular system evaluation, 8–10
Catheterization, postoperative, 150
Cefazolin, 13, 43
Cefotetan, 13
Cefoxitin, 139
Cellulitis, pelvic, 143
　postoperative, 159–160
Chest radiographs, 5–6
Chlamydia trachomatis, 133, 134
Cholecystectomy, 126
Clindamycin, 140
Clotting mechanism, defects of, 79–80, 80f
Colporrhaphy, 121–122
Concomitant surgery, 115–128
　abdominoplasty, 127
　appendectomy, 125–126
　cholecystectomy, 126
　colporrhaphy, 121–122
　liposuction, 127–128
　oophorectomy, 115–121
　reteropubic urethropexy, 124–125
　vaginal vault management, 122–123
Congestive heart failure, 9
Constipation, postoperative, 154
Controversial techniques, 103–112
　enterocele and vault prolapse prevention, 109
　luteinizing hormone-releasing hormone agonists, 106–108
　outpatient vaginal hysterectomy, 108–109
　peritoneal closure, 110
　salpingo-oophorectomy, 111–112
　uterine morcellation, 103–105
　vaginal cuff closure, 109–110
　vasoconstrictivity agent use, 110–111
Coronary artery disease, 9
Crystalloid solution, and hemorrhage, 84
Culdoplasty, 112–123
Cultural aspects, and hysterectomy response, 172
Cystoscopy, and bladder fistulas, 43
Cystotomy, 187

D

Danazol, 186
Demel technique, 65, 65f
Depression, 169–173

Diabetes, postoperative medication reinstitution, 152–153
Diagnostic procedures, 4–6
Diet, postoperative, 153–154
Dilation and curettage, in endometrial hyperplasia, 23
Dissection, operative, and ovarian remnant syndrome, 187–188, 187f–189f
Disseminated intravascular coagulation, 80–81
Doxycycline, 139
Dressings, abdominal, 154
Drug fever, 160
Dyspareunia, 178

E

Elective hysterectomy, 23
Electrocardiogram, 6
Electrolytes, postoperative, 150
Embolism, pulmonary, 156
Emotional issues. *See* Psychosocial aspects
Emphysema, 8
Endloop technique, and oophorectomies, 112
Endocarditis, bacterial, 13
Endometrial sampling, 23
Endometriosis, 21–22
　and laparoscopic-assisted vaginal hysterectomy, 197, 198
Endoscopic staples, and laparoscopic-assisted vaginal hysterectomy, 194t, 194–196
Enterocele, posthysterectomy, 109
Enterococcus faecalis, 36
Epidemiology, 18–20
Epinephrine, and blood loss, 110–111
Escherichia coli, 36
Estrogen therapy
　and ovarian remnant syndrome, 186
　postsurgical, 153
　and thromboembolism, 10
Exposure, and hemorrhage prevention, 86

F

Fears, patient, 3
Feedings, postoperative, 153–154
Financial advantages, of antibiotic prophylaxis use, 40, 42

Fistulas
　bladder, 52–59
　　abdominal closure of, 59
　　diagnosis of, 53–54
　　large fistula repair, 57f, 57–58, 58f
　　Latzko technique, 55–57, 56f
　　local tissue grafts, 59
　　repair timing, 55
　　surgical considerations, 55
　　symptoms, 53
　　transvaginal closure, 58t, 58–59
　genitourinary, 155
　small bowel, 70–71
Fitz-Hugh-Curtis syndrome, 136
Flashback incidents, posthysterectomy, 171–172
Fluids, postoperative, 150
Follicle-stimulating hormone, and ovarian remnant syndrome, 185–186
Fresh frozen plasma, and hemorrhage, 84

G

Gambee closure, 69, 71, 71f–74f, 73
Gastrointestinal complications, postoperative, 158–159
Gastrointestinal tract evaluation, 10–11
Gentamicin, 140
GnRH, in leiomyomata, 21
Goals of hysterectomy, 29–31
Guaiac test, 5
Gynecological complaints. *See also* Psychosocial aspects emotional issues as underlying cause, 164–169

H

Heaney technique, 31
Hematoma, infundibulopelvic ligament, 88
Hemisection, and uterine morcellation, 103
Hemoglobin determination, 5
Hemogram, 149
Hemophilia, 82
Hemorrhage, 79–99
　bleeding diathesis diagnosis, 83
　bleeding disorders
　　acquired, 80–82
　　congenital, 82–83

Hemorrhage [cont.]
  clotting mechanism defects, 79–80
  coagulation systems, 80f
  intraoperative bleeding, 83–98. See also Bleeding, intraoperative
  posthysterectomy, 98–99, 157
  replacement formulas, 84
  surgical bleeding categories, 79
Heparin, postoperative, 152
Historical aspects, 18
History taking, 3–4
Hormone replacement regimens, and oophorectomy, 119
Hospital discharge, 160, 161t
Hot flashes, 184
Hyperplasia, endometrial, 22–23
Hypertension, 9–10
  postoperative, 157
Hypogastric artery, divisions of, 85t
Hypogastric artery ligation, 89–95
  anatomy, 91
  collateral circulation, 91
  complications and efficacy, 93, 95
  hemodynamics, 91–92
  indications for, 90t
  surgical technique, 92f–97f, 92–93
Hypotension, postoperative, 157
Hypothermia, and blood transfusions, 81
Hysteria. See Briquet's syndrome

I

Ileus, paralytic, 158
Incisions, vaginal, care of, 154
Incontinence surgery, 124–125
Indications, 20–23
  cancer, 22
  endometrial hyperplasia, 22–23
  endometriosis, 21–22
  leiomyomata, 20–21
  prolapse, 22
Infection, 23
  distant, 42
  in pelvic inflammatory disease, 133–134
  risk factors for, 36–37
  wound, 159
Informed consent, 1–3
  ethical components of, 2
  and surgical approach choice, 29
Infundibulopelvic ligament hematoma, 88

Intramyometrial coring, and uterine morcellation, 104
Intravenous pyelogram, 11–12

K

Kegel exercises, and urogenital prolapse, 22

L

Laboratory tests, 5
Laparoscopic-assisted vaginal hysterectomy, 191–198
  history and results of, 191–194
  multifire endoscopic staples and, 194–196
  role of, 196–198
Laparoscopy. See also Laparoscopic-assisted vaginal hysterectomy
  and adnexal pathology, 30–31
  and cancer, 198
  and endometriosis, 21
  and ovarian remnant syndrome, 185
  and pelvic inflammatory disease, 137–138
Laparotomy, and pelvic inflammatory disease, 140–142
Large bowel injuries, 73–75. See also Bowel injuries
Lash procedure, and uterine morcellation, 104
Latzko partial colpocleisis technique, 55–57, 56f
Leiomyomata
  as indication for hysterectomy, 20–21
  luteinizing hormone-releasing hormone agonists and, 106, 106t
Leuprolide acetate therapy, 107–108
Ligation, hypogastric artery. See Hypogastric artery ligation
Liposuction, concurrent, 127–128
Liver function tests, 5
Luteinizing hormone-releasing hormone agonists, 106–108
  data summary, 107t
  effects on leiomyomata uteri, 106t

M

Mammography, 5
Martius technique, 59

Medication reinstitution, postoperative, 152–153
Menopausal symptoms, and oophorectomy, 119
Mental health. *See* Psychological aspects
Military antishock trousers, 97–98
Mitral valve prolapse, 9
Mixter clamp, 92f–95f, 93
Morcellation, uterine, during vaginal hysterectomy
   combination of methods, 104
   hemisection/bivalving, 103
   lash procedure/intramyometrial coring, 104
   procedural tips, 105t
   safety of, 104–106
   wedge morcellation, 104
Myocardial infarctions, 9
Myomectomy, for leiomyomata, 21

N

Nausea, postoperative, 153
Neisseria gonorrhoeae, 133, 134

O

Obesity, and pulmonary complications, 7
Obstetric emergencies, 23
Obstruction
   large bowel, 158
   small bowel, 158
Oophorectomy, 115–121
   advantages of, 117–118
   disadvantages of, 119–120
   incidence of, 116–117
   psychological impact of, 177
   technique of, 120–121
   at vaginal hysterectomy, 30, 111–112
Opiates, and pain control, 150
Oral contraceptives, 10
Osteoporosis, and oophorectomy, 119–120
Outpatient vaginal hysterectomy, 108–109
Ovarian cancer, and oophorectomy, 117–118
Ovarian remnant syndrome, 183–189
   ancillary tests for, 184–186
   clinical presentation, 184
   complications, 189
   etiology of, 184
   incidence of, 183
   operative findings, 188
   treatment, 186–188
      nonoperative, 186
      operative procedures, 187–188
Ovaries, removal of. *See* Oophorectomy

P

Pain, pelvic
   and laparoscopic-assisted vaginal hysterectomy, 198
   and ovarian remnant syndrome, 184
Pain control, postoperative, 150
Papanicolaou smear, 5
Patient education, and surgical approach choice, 29
Pelvic adhesive disease, and laparoscopic-assisted vaginal hysterectomy, 197
Pelvic arteriovenous malformation, 23
Pelvic bleeding
   anatomy of, 84–85
   physiology of, 85
Pelvic inflammatory disease, 133–143
   atypical salpingitis, 136
   chronic, 136
   diagnosis of, 134–136
   Fitz-Hugh-Curtis syndrome, 136
   hysterectomy and, 142–143
   laparoscopy and, 137–138
   pathophysiology of, 133–134
   related conditions, 136
   surgical management, 140–142
   treatment of, 138–140, 139t
Pelvic packs, 88–89
Pelvic relaxation, 123
Peritoneal closure, 110
Pessary, and urogenital prolapse, 22
Physical examination, 3–4
Platelet disorders
   acquired, 82
   congenital, 82–83
Pneumonia, 156
Posthysterectomy, bleeding. *See* Bleeding
Postoperative care, 147–161
   ambulation, 154
   bladder drainage, 150–152
   cardiovascular complications, 157–158
   discharge from hospital, 160, 161t

Postoperative care [cont.]
  drug fever, 160
  feedings, 153–154
  fluids and electrolytes, 150
  gastrointestinal complications, 158–159
  hemogram, 149
  medication reinstitution, 152–153
  pain control, 150
  pelvic cellulitis, 159–160
  postoperative note format, 148t
  postoperative orders format, 148t
  recovery room care, 147–148
  respiratory complications, 155–156
  transfusions, 149
  urinary complications, 155
  wound care, 154
  wound complications, 159
Premenstrual syndrome, and oophorectomy, 118
Preoperative considerations, 1–13
  antibiotic usage, 12–13
  diagnostic procedures, 4–6
  history taking, 3–4
  informed consent, 1–3
  physical examination, 3–4
  psychological aspects, 3
  systems evaluation, 6–12
Procoagulant disorders
  acquired, 82
  congenital, 82
Progesterone therapy
  and endometrial hyperplasia, 23
  and ovarian remnant syndrome, 186
Prolapse, urogenital, 22, 30
Prophylactic sacrospinous fixation, of vagina, 123
Psychological changes. See also Psychosocial aspects
  posthysterectomy, 169–176
Psychosocial aspects, 3, 163–178
  abdominal hysterectomy effects, 177–178
  anxiety, 169–173
  behavior problems, 173–174
  Briquet's syndrome, 164–169
  depression, 169–173
  dyspareunia and, 178
  historic perspective, 164
  oophorectomy effects, 177
  sexual dysfunction, 174–176
  sterilization impact and, 176–177
  supravaginal uterine amputation effects, 177–178

Pulmonary disease, 7–8
Pulmonary function tests, 6–7
Puncture injury, bowel, 68f, 68–69
Pyelography, and ovarian remnant syndrome, 185, 185f

Q

Quality assurance process, and indication assessment, 19–20

R

Radiotherapy, and ovarian remnant syndrome, 186
Rebound abdominal tenderness, 159
Recovery room care, 147–148
Replacement formulas, for hemorrhage, 84
Respiratory complications, postoperative, 155–156
Respiratory failure, postoperative, 156
Respiratory system evaluation, 6–8
Retropubic urethropexy, 124–125

S

Salpingitis. See also Pelvic inflammatory disease
  acute, 135
  atypical, 136
Salpingo-oophorectomy. See Oophorectomy
Sex steroid production, and oophorectomy, 119–120
Sexual abuse, and posthysterectomy emotional problems, 172
Sexual dysfunction, after hysterectomy, 174–176
Sexual intercourse
  painful after hysterectomy, 178
  and postoperative wound care, 154
Sexually transmitted disease, and pelvic inflammatory disease, 140
Small bowel injuries, 70–73. See also Bowel injuries
Smoking, and pulmonary complications, 7
Somatization disorder, 164–169
Stapling instruments, in bowel injury closure, 73

Sterilization, 23
  adverse psychological reactions and, 176–177
Storage pool disease, 83
Subtotal hysterectomy, 28
Surgical approach, choice of, 27–32
Surgical technique, and prevention of bleeding, 86–87

T

Tears, bowel, 69f, 69–70
Thromboasthenia, 83
Thromboembolism, 10
Thrombophlebitis, 157–158
Thrombosis, deep venous, 157
Tissue grafts, and bladder fistulas, 59
Transfusion, 149
  bleeding secondary to, 81–82
Transureteroureterostomy, 66
Trichomonas vaginalis, 36
Tuboovarian abscess formation, 134

U

Ultrasonography, and ovarian remnant syndrome, 184–185
Ureteral injuries, 59–66
  conditions associated with, 60t
  intraoperative diagnosis and repair, 60–62, 61f
  prevention, 59–60
  types of repair, 63t
  unrecognized injury, 62–66
    diagnosis of, 62
    repair timing, 62–63
    surgical considerations, 63
    ureteroneocystostomy, 63–65, 64f, 65t
    ureteroureterostomies, 65–66, 66f
Ureteral injury, postoperative, 155
Ureteroneocystostomy, 63–65, 64f
  Boari-Ockerblad flap, 64f
  Demel technique, 65f
Ureteroureterostomies, 65–66, 66f
Urinalysis, 5
Urinary complications, postoperative, 155
Urinary tract evaluation, 11–12
Urinary tract infections, postoperative, 155

V

Vaginal cuff closure, 109–110
Vaginal hysterectomy
  benefits of, 27–28
  contraindications to, 28–29
  psychiatric aspects of, 177–178
  techniques of, 31–32
Vaginal vault management, 122–123
Valvular heart disease, 9
Vasocontrictivity agent use, 110–111
Vault prolapse, vaginal, 109
Vomiting, postoperative, 153
Von Willebrand's disease, 82

W

Walking, postoperative, 154
Wedge morcellation, 104
Wiskott-Aldrich syndrome, 82
Wound care, postoperative, 154
Wound complications, postoperative, 159